BALTIMORE CITY HOSPITALS - 1904
from the 1904 Baltimore City Directory

Baltimore Eye, Ear and Throat Charity Hospital*
    625 West Franklin Street
Church Home and Infirmary
    Broadway near Fairmount Avenue
City Hospital and Dispensary* (connected with the College of Physicians and Surgeons)
    Calvert and Saratoga Streets
City Hospital Annex (for colored patients)
    112 E. Saratoga Street
City Hospital for the Insane (Bayview)*
    Eastern Avenue ext.
Emergency Toxocological Hospital*
    Franklin Square, nw corner Calhoun and Fayette Streets
Greater Free Hospital for Children
    27 N. Carey Street
Hebrew Hospital and Asylum*
    Monument Street and Hopkins Avenue
Hospital for Consumptives of Maryland
    Eudowood Station
Hospital for the Relief of Crippled and Deformed Children*
    Charles Street near 20th Street
Hospital of the Good Samaritan
    1030 McCulloh Street
Hospital of the Woman's Medical College
    1030 McCulloh Street
Hospital for the Women of Maryland*
    Lafayette Avenue and John Street
Johns Hopkins Hospital and Infirmary*
    Broadway and Monument Street
Maryland General Hospital*
    Madison and Linden Aves.
Maryland Homeopathic Hospital
    1122 N. Mount Street
Maternity (Lying-In) Hospital
    115 W. Lombard Street
Nursery and Children's Hospital
    Schroeder and Franklin Streets
Presbyterian Eye, Ear and Throat Hospital
    1007 E. Baltimore Street
Provident Hospital (colored)
    413-415 W. Biddle Street
St. Agnes Sanitarium and Dispensary*
    Caton and Wilkens Aves.
St. Joseph's Hospital and Free Dispensary*
    Caroline and Hoffman Streets
Union Protestant Infirmary*
    1514-1522 Division Street
United States Marine Hospital
    Remington Avenue nr. 31st Street
University Hospital (formerly Baltimore Infirmary)*
    Lombard and Greene Streets

*Denotes a hospital still in operation in 2004 - may be a different name and address

BALTIMORE CITY HOSPITALS - 2004
From the 2004 Greater Baltimore Yellow Pages

Bon Secours Baltimore Health Center
 2000 W. Baltimore Street
University Specialty Hospital
 611 S. Charles Street
Good Samaritan Hospital of Maryland
 5601 Loch Raven Blvd.
Harbor Hospital Center
 3001 S. Hanover Street
The Johns Hopkins Hospital*
 600 N. Wolfe Street
Johns Hopkins Bayview Medical Center*
 4940 Eastern Avenue
Maryland General Hospital*
 827 Linden Avenue
Mercy Medical Center*
 301 St. Paul Place
Mt. Washington Pediatric Hospital
 1708 W. Rogers Avenue
St. Agnes Healthcare*
 900 Caton Avenue
Sinai Hospital*
 2401 W. Belvedere
Union Memorial Hospital*
 201 E. University Pkwy.
University of Maryland Medical Systems*
 419 Redwood Street
Kennedy Krieger Institute
 707 N. Broadway
James Lawrence Kernan Hospital*
 2200 Kernan Drive
Keswick Multi-Care Center
 700 West 40th Street
Levindale Hebrew Geriatric Center and Hospital
 2434 W. Belvedere Avenue
VA Maryland Health Care System
 10 N. Greene Street

*Denotes a hospital that was in operation in 1904 - may be a different name and address

SPECIAL ACKNOWLEDGMENTS

The Baltimore City Medical Society expresses its deep appreciation to those whose generosity made the publication of this book a reality:

Allan D. Jensen, M.D.
Anil Uberoi, M.D.
Reed A. Winston, M.D.

Anne S. Barone, M.D.
Marshall S. Bedine, M.D.
Beverly A. Collins, M.D.
Tyler C. Cymet, D.O.
Worth B. Daniels, Jr., M.D.
John Burling De Hoff, M.D.
Dr. and Mrs. Donald H. Dembo
Willarda V. Edwards, M.D.
James "Seamus" Flynn, M.D.
Maurice B. Furlong, M.D.
Moges Gebremariam, M.D.
F. Michael Gloth, III, M.D.
Eve J. Higginbotham, M.D.
Charles F. Hobelmann, Jr., M.D.
Thomas E. Hunt, Jr., M.D.
Jeffrey R. Kaplan, M.D.
Ferdinand Leacock, M.D.
Hiroshi Nakazawa, M.D.
Anthony J. Raneri, M.D.
Michael A. Randolph, M.D.
Anuradha Reddy, M.D.
Gary L. Rosenberg, M.D.
John T. Thompson, M.D.
Levi Watkins, M.D.
Karl H. Weaver, M.D.
Jos W. Zebley, III, M.D.

"...to advance the ethical practice of medicine and improve the quality of health care..."

The Baltimore City Medical Society

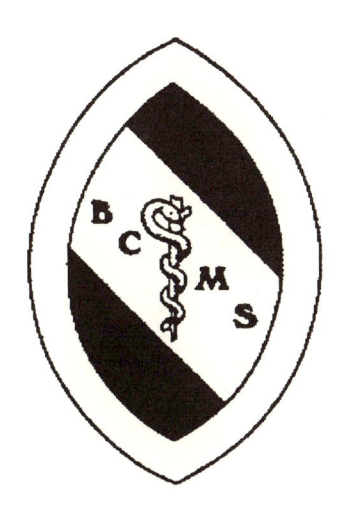

A History

by Ron and Pat Pilling

Published on the Occasion of the Centenary of the
Modern Baltimore City Medical Society
as a component of the
Medical and Chirurgical Faculty of Maryland

2004
American Literary Press
Baltimore

The Baltimore City Medical Society: A History

Copyright © 2004 The Baltimore City Medical Society

All rights reserved under International and Pan-American copyright conventions. No part of this book may be reproduced, stored in a retrieval system, or transmitted in any form, electronic, mechanical, or other means, now known or hereafter invented, without written permission of the author. Address all inquiries to the Baltimore City Medical Society.

Library of Congress
Cataloging-in-Publication Data
ISBN 1-56167-867-8

FIRST EDITION

Published by

American Literary Press, Inc.
8019 Belair Road, Suite 10
Baltimore, Maryland 21236

Manufactured in the United States of America

MARTIN O'MALLEY
Mayor
250 City Hall
Baltimore, Maryland 21202

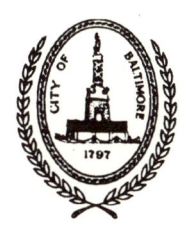

May 2004

A MESSAGE FROM MAYOR MARTIN O'MALLEY

Dear Friends,

Baltimore is known around the world and across the country as America's leading health care center. People who have the means to go anywhere in the world for their health care needs choose to come to Baltimore to receive the best medical treatment available anywhere. While we often may think our city is best known for the Inner Harbor or Camden Yards, it is our medical institutions that have the widest global reach.

For nearly two centuries, the work of our greatest medical institutions has kept millions of people around the world safe from illness and harm by pioneering new research, using knowledge and expertise in hospitals and care facilities home and abroad, and educating future leaders in the science and practice of the global defense of human life. Due to these institutions, supported by an enviable network of community hospitals and health care centers, Baltimore medical professionals' accomplishments are legendary.

These same caregivers have organized themselves into professional societies for equally as long, and it is fitting that the Baltimore City Medical Society should look back on its history with satisfaction. Its advocacy, and that of its individual members, in the area of public health has resulted in clean drinking water, safe and healthy milk for Baltimore's children, and improvements in public hygiene that put an end to the periodic epidemics which devastated

Baltimore neighborhoods a century ago. The Society's public outreach work has educated both laymen and professionals, making us all better consumers of, and providers of, quality health care services. It is a legacy of which you, as a member or a potential member, of the Society can be proud.

Our future as a pinnacle people, as a pinnacle society, and the future of leadership of this increasingly smaller world, will be determined by the number of smart hands and healing hearts we can extend openly to our neighbors throughout the world. I would like to congratulate the members of the medical community of Baltimore City on the centenary of the Baltimore City Medical Society. Together, I hope we will continue to work toward serving and healing our neighbors at home and abroad.

Sincerely,

Mayor

FOREWORD

Henry Ford said history is more or less bunk. Voltaire *may* have said history is a pack of lies we tell on the dead. With that in mind, this volume has been prepared for your entertainment and occasional information. Fact and fancy are often inseparable for contemporaries. How much less for us. In 1995, on the 50th anniversary of V-E Day, Mrs. Hunt and I were walking behind a group of teenagers and overheard one exclaim that her grandfather had served in World War II. A companion asked whether that was before or after the Civil War. Looking back, we may think on our own estates and wonder how the future will view us.

Baltimore City Medical Society is celebrating our centennial in 2004, as it was in 1904 that the structure as we know it was laid down. Our beginnings, however, date back to the first meeting on December 15, 1788 of The Medical Society of Baltimore, at which Dr. Elisha Hall spoke on the necessity for regulations on the practice of "physick." This volume traces our highs and lows over the intervening 216 years. So think not inconsiderately of our medical forebears most of whom, we hope, done their durndest.

Ron and Pat Pilling, the Past Presidents Committee chaired by Beverly A. Collins, M.D., and Lisa B. Williams, Executive Director of the Baltimore City Medical Society, have made much effort to assure the purity of this product which surely has full measure of false negatives and positives.

-Thomas E. Hunt, Jr., M.D.
Historian, Baltimore City Medical Society
April 19, 2004

TABLE OF CONTENTS

Welcome from Mayor Martin O'Malley
Foreword by Dr. Thomas E. Hunt, Jr.

The Chronology

The First Century of Medical Societies in Baltimore	3
The Medical Profession in Baltimore Enters the 20th Century	25
The Baltimore City Medical Society Enters the Post-World War II Years	47
"Every Physician will have to become a lobbyist" 1960 - 2004	69

The Missions

Medical Ethics	93
Public Health and Sanitation in Baltimore	111
Scientific Sections and Sessions: The Society's Role in Professional Education	129
The Baltimore City Medical Society and the Economics of Healthcare	135
Nostrums and Drugs, Legal and Otherwise	159
The Baltimore City Medical Society Auxiliary and the Baltimore City Medical Society Foundation	171
Presidents of Baltimore City Medical Societies	179
Bibliography	217
Acknowledgments	223
Baltimore City Commissioners of Health	224

"Every boy in the street gang knows the joy of sharing, of being a member of the gang, and every Doctor who belongs to a state or city society has a similar pleasure of sharing, in helping to cherish the ideals of the group and especially when the aims of a group are so definite and appealing, the influence upon every member of the group cannot help but be strongly felt and that gives to each member of the group an honest sense of security."

-Dr. William Henry Welch
at a meeting of the Baltimore City Medical Society
April 6, 1926

"What does the Faculty mean to its members? One always feels sorry for the man who asks this question. If he were interested, he would know. The member gets out of it just what he puts into it, - and more, in proportion to his loyalty to the profession and to the Society...the Library...Physicians Defense is of more value in money than the entire amount of dues. Protection against foolish and destructive legislation; the value of organization, scientific and professional; public health propaganda; social, educational, political, economic and historical censorship...Were it not for the medical societies the quacks...would swamp us...They do not hesitate to spend their money; we do."

"Let us put this proposition across with a bang. Don't be a 'Poor me!' or a 'Who me?' but a 'Count on me.'"

-Dr. Lewellys F. Barker
at a meeting of the Baltimore City Medical Society
April 6, 1926

"Why join a Society? You may not get everything you want working from the inside, but you get nothing when you try to work from the outside."

-Dr. Roland E. Smoot
from a February, 2004 interview

"Let us now sum up some of the advantages of the study of medical history:

1. It teaches what and how to investigate.

2. It is the best antidote we know against egotism, error and despondency.

3. It increases knowledge, gratifies natural and laudable curiosity, broadens the view and strengthens the judgement.

4. It is a rich mine from which may be brought to light many neglected or overlooked discoveries of value.

5. It furnishes the stimulus of high ideals which we poor, weak mortals need to have ever before us; It teaches our students to venerate what is good, to cherish our best traditions, and strengthen the common bonds of the profession.

6. It is the fulfillment of a duty - that of cherishing the memories, the virtues, the achievements of a class which has benefitted the world as no other has, and of which we may feel proud that we are members."

- Eugene F. Cordell, M.D.
1903

"FOR PROFESSIONAL ADVANCEMENT, THE DIFFUSION OF KNOWLEDGE, AND THE CULTIVATION OF FRIENDLY RELATIONS..."

The First Century of Medical Societies in Baltimore

From the windows in the dome of the Exchange Building looking southwest, one could, in early 1866, clearly see the remnants of General Benjamin Butler's Fort Federal Hill, from which a phalanx of cannon glowered down upon the city of Baltimore throughout the duration of the Civil War. Earthworks remained, as did the two-story barracks and the watchtower. Only the blue-and red uniformed Duryea Zouaves, the soldiers of the 7th New York Regiment and all the other troops in blue had decamped.

The last thing needed by the eight colleagues who gathered in the Exchange office of Baltimore City Health Commissioner Gerard Edwin Morgan, M.D., on February 26th, was a reminder of those terrible four years. Each had seen the worst that war could devise in an era when Napoleonic tactics had been brutally surpassed by the technology of killing. Each of the eight gentlemen still had the pungent odor of the field hospital in his nostrils as he settled into Commissioner Morgan's office, for each had served as either an assistant surgeon or a surgeon in the Union Army.

It was imperative, the group agreed, that the horrible lessons of the war, as well as the advances in medicine that were purchased at the expense of more than 618,000 lives and even more limbs, not be forgotten. Something positive, something redeeming must be part of the legacy of the struggle. The American Civil War had, after all, taught the medical community valuable lessons about ambulance services, surgical techniques, public health and hospital organization. As the eight surgeons recalled their experiences they concluded that the impulse to form a new professional society for the physicians of Baltimore was a good one. The groundwork for the Baltimore Medical Association was laid that day in February, 1866, and there is a direct connection between that organization and the modern Baltimore City Medical Society.

Among the eight founders, Dr. Morgan served as an Assistant Surgeon for the United States Volunteers in 1861, returning to civilian life before the surrender was signed in 1865. Dr. James H. Currey served with the 3rd Maryland Infantry Volunteers through the summer of 1862. This duty placed him in a field hospital during the battle of Cedar Mountain, in which there were 1,400 Union casualties, as well as on the field at the Battle of Antietam, the bloodiest day in United States military history. From 1863 until the end of the war, Dr. Currey was Post Surgeon at Fort McHenry. The fort served as a prisoner of war Camp, and following the Battle of Gettysburg (the beginning of Dr. Currey's posting there) it held nearly seven thousand prisoners.

"The End of the Medical Middle Ages"

United States Surgeon General William Hammond used that phrase to describe the condition of health care at the outbreak of the American Civil War in 1861. American physicians had little knowledge of the work of Pasteur and because an understanding of infection and the link between sanitation and the spread of disease was lacking, surgery was septic. Even thorough handwashing between operations was unknown, although considering the quality of water with which surgeons had to work (usually lukewarm and bloody minutes into a battle) its effectiveness would have been in doubt.

Treatment was barbaric by modern standards. The Medical Director of the Army of the Potomac, Dr. Jonathan Letterman (famed for his creation of a modern ambulance service) reacted to criticism of his doctors' propensity to amputate by saying that, if anything, doctors were too conservative in removing arms and legs. A good surgeon could complete an amputation in ten minutes, and time was a scarce resource in the field hospital. This was much more expeditious than trying to reconstruct shattered bone and torn flesh, which would in all likelihood have later required amputation anyway.

For every soldier who died in battle, two succumbed to disease. Bowel complaints were treated with opium or the dreaded "blue mass" - a mixture of mercury and chalk. Respiratory problems were treated with opium, or quinine and mustard plasters. Soldiers dealt with "camp itch" by immersing themselves in a poke root and water solution. Blood poisoning, tetanus and gangrene almost always meant a death sentence.

Yet from the chaos of the field surgical tent and the abysmal condition of churches-turned-hospitals in every small town in the battle zone, huge advances were made which dramatically improved civilian medical care after the war. The copious notes made by doctors during the war were compiled into *The Medical and Surgical History of the War of the Rebellion* between 1870 and 1888. These experiences helped post-war physicians treat dysentery, diarrhea, typhoid and malaria. By the close of the war, doctors understood that enforcing minimal sanitary standards would reduce infection and slow epidemics. Experience in treating gangrene led to the discovery and use of bromine.

The most significant improvements in medical care resulted from hospital

THE BALTIMORE CITY MEDICAL SOCIETY - A History

reorganization and the delivery of sick and wounded to hospitals. In 1861, both civilian and military hospitals were organized on an as-needed basis, understaffed and unsanitary. Hospitals were single buildings with no differentiation based on illness, so many failed to survive their stays not because of what brought them to the hospital in the first place, but because they contracted something someone else brought. By war's end, hospitals were divided into wards which stemmed the spread of disease. Also, the idea of professional nursing was born when Dorothea Dix was appointed Superintendent of the United States Nursing Corps in 1861. Finally, field hospitals moved from filthy barns and makeshift outbuildings to larger, well-ventilated tents and more permanent centers for treatment and convalescence.

By September, 1862, the Army of the Potomac had adopted Doctor Jonathan Letterman's ambulance plan. The plan brought organization to the task of removing the wounded from the battlefield and getting them to a doctor's care as quickly as possible. The number of stretcher bearers per ambulance was standardized, and an ambulance corps created to move in concert with advancing forces. This was a vast improvement over the earlier system, military or civilian, which was haphazard and operated by men with no experience whatsoever except the ability to drive a team. The Letterman Ambulance Plan became the foundation for hundreds of civilian ambulance systems after the war.

Even a museum was established that would be a valuable resource to civilian practitioners. The "Army Medical Museum" was a repository of medical and surgical specimens, including some celebrity specimens like the leg of Major General Dan Sickles, lost to an artillery round at Gettysburg. The collection is now at the Smithsonian Institution.

A total of 40 surgeons lost their lives in the Union Army alone during the war. Those who returned and were still able to practice brought with them experience which, while costly, was priceless in building the road to modern medicine.

Doctors George H. Dare and John Neff served as assistant surgeons with the Army of the Potomac from 1861 until Lee's surrender. Dr. Charles Hyland Jones was the Acting Assistant Surgeon, US Volunteers, in charge of Jarvis Hospital from 1861 until the hospital was closed in 1865. Jarvis Hospital was a 1700-bed military hospital at the western end of Baltimore Street, on the confiscated estate of General George H. Steuart, CSA.

One of the veterans in the Exchange that February, 1866 day had seen the other side of the war, as a prisoner. Dr. Lewis M. Eastman, Sr. was taken prisoner in August, 1862 in the Kanawha Valley in what would become West Virginia, where he was serving in General George McClellan's Army of the Potomac. He was exchanged and served out the war with the 1st US Cavalry.

The two remaining places at the first meeting of the Baltimore Medical Association were also filled by Civil War veterans. Dr. A.A. White was a surgeon with 3rd Infantry and 8th Infantry, US Volunteers from 1861 until 1863 and Dr. William G. Smull was an assistant surgeon for the entire war.

On March 6, 1866, the founders again convened at the Baltimore City Department of Health and drew up a Constitution and By-Laws, adopting the name "Baltimore Medical Association." Dr. Morgan was named President and an office established at 47 Calvert Street. This was the address of the Medical and Chirurgical Faculty of Maryland until 1867. Part professional society, part social club, the Baltimore Medical Association was created to foster "professional advancement, the diffusion of knowledge, and the cultivation of friendly relations."

A small booklet, bound in hand-marbled end papers, dated 1866 and printed by Frederick A. Hanzsche, 234 W. Baltimore Street, is still in the possession of the Baltimore City Medical Society. It contains the Constitution and By-Laws of the Baltimore Medical Association as drawn up by seven of the association's earliest members. From these first statements of the organization's mission and the guidelines by which it was created and operated, a portrait of a group of dedicated professionals emerges. They were "...persuaded of the advantages which a well regulated professional intercourse, may render to the Medical faculty in the diffusion of knowledge, the establishment of salutary rules of etiquette, and the cultivation of friendly sentiments" in establishing standards to govern their conduct of business. They also agreed to follow the code of ethics adopted by the American Medical Association in 1847.

Quickly dispatching the customary housekeeping responsibilities of the Association's officers, the original Constitution lays out a plan for applicant admission and a committee structure. The "Committee of Honor" was charged with the responsibility of carefully examining every applicant's fitness for membership, taking into consideration "all matters relating to Professional Etiquette" and sketching a mechanism by which complaints about a member's character were to be made.

What exactly might have disqualified a physician for Association membership? The Constitution is precise on this point: "Giving a certificate of the efficacy of any secret medicine...Receiving a percentage or any other remuneration from druggists on prescriptions, or being in any manner interested in the sale of drugs

THE BALTIMORE CITY MEDICAL SOCIETY - A History

and medicines...disobedience of the Code of Ethics."

Membership required that a physician prepare periodic lectures and discussions to be presented to the group. A Committee on Lectures and Discussions was established to propose topics of interest and enlist members to conduct the evenings' talks, "consistent with the objects of the Association." The Executive Committee acted as a combined nominating committee and auditor. Officers and Board members held their positions for just 12 months, with elections taking place in February of each calendar year.

After receiving the approval of the Committee of Honor, an applicant had only to pay the $1.00 initiation fee and his or her first year's dues of $2.00 to complete the admission process. Providing the dues were kept current, and the member avoided reprimand for violating the AMA's Code of Ethics, he could continue to enjoy the benefits of membership in the Baltimore Medical Association and attend the semi-monthly meetings. The Order of Business, as described in the By-Laws, acted as an agenda for each meeting. Clearly, the priority of the organization was the dissemination of knowledge and the sharing of professional experience, for those functions precede the normal administrative committee reports and general business. Following the delivery of the lecture, time was allotted for the discussion of current cases by members. To conclude each meeting, a topic for the lecture of the subsequent session was chosen by the member who was to deliver it, and approved by the members present.

There being no Sergeant at Arms among the Officers, rules for addressing the group were specified in the By-Laws. "In debate the member shall rise from his seat and address the Chair; and shall confine himself to the subject under discussion, avoiding personal reflections or sarcastic remarks. For violation of this rule, any member may be called to order by the President or any member, and shall take his seat until the question of order shall have been decided."

The Baltimore Medical Association grew rapidly until by 1883 there were 76 paid members. Dr. G. Lane Taneyhill, who presided over this Association in 1874, delivered in 1881 an address entitled "Historical Sketches of the Medical Societies of Baltimore, Md., from 1730 to 1880." His talk was part of the state Faculty's celebration of the 150th anniversary of Baltimore, and in it Dr. Taneyhill noted the importance of the Civil War in medical history: "The late war was a great dividing line, and marked the vast social and intellectual change in our midst. A new and better era dawned upon us, and the 'Baltimore Medical Association' was the first fruits of the new birth. It was the offspring of a necessity which had to be provided for; It has fully met the want and, as the *pioneer* of the present local medical organizations, deserves the gratitude, respect and support of the profession."

Baltimore's First Medical Societies

The Baltimore Medical Association, while being the "pioneer" of organizations that followed, was not the first of its kind in the city's history. Clamor for an organization to regulate the practice of medicine in Baltimore and statewide arose as early as 1785, when an unnamed correspondent to the *Maryland Journal and Baltimore Daily Advertiser*, in the November 25th issue, wrote:

> "I fully intended to write you on the Subject of a medical Establishment, but a variety of Matters has constantly deranged my Ideas...I am really provoked by the Credulity of the People in this Vicinity, in trusting to, consequently in supporting a Number of villainous Quacks, who are imposing on them daily. I have taken some Pains to expose them...If a Number of respectable Physicians would join in a Petition to the Legislature, praying that some Mode of licensing Practitioners in Physic and Surgery may be adopted, I am of the Opinion that it would certainly be attended to."

Responses were printed regularly in the same newspaper. On December 23rd a citizen (signed "Anonymous") echoed the first letter by opining that "There is no difference between a man who offers you a dose, uncertain what its effects may be, solely for a premium, and one who presents his pistol to your breast, and demands your money, except the first is the most to be dreaded of the two: The highwayman may be satisfied with your purse, while the obdurate heart of the quack, insensible to every finer sensation, continues to thirst after lucre, even at the expence of your life."

This same correspondent continued, offering a plan by which the General Assembly would grant incorporation to a group of physicians whose responsibility it would be to judge the competence of those proposing to enter the profession, and to "license such as may be found qualified."

Yet another, signed "A Citizen", wrote on the same day in 1785, "A

Medicinal Society will hereafter be a convenient medium through which the diseases incident to our climate, and constitution, may be made public...Every practitioner is or ought to be capable of relating the history of any disorder...Such facts, after the Society's evaluation, may be published for the benefit of such as may desire to improve...A Medicinal Society will be a further introduction to a school of Physic and Surgery, both of which we are destitute."

Several years passed before the *Federal Gazette and Baltimore Commercial Daily Advertiser* could report on December 26, 1788 the creation of the "Medical Society of Baltimore", probably the first formal society of professional physicians in the city's short history. The founders were Drs. Charles Friedrich Wiesenthal and Frederick Dalcho. Wiesenthal was the first medical professor of significance in Baltimore, teaching prospective doctors from his residence at Gay and Fayette Streets. He served during the American Revolution as Superintendent for the Manufacture of Saltpetre, and as surgeon to troops from Maryland. Dalcho was a student of Wiesenthal.

Dr. Wiesenthal had already established himself as the foremost physician in the state. During the Revolutionary War, he laid out innovative plans for medical evacuation from the battlefield and for hospitalization. Calling for "flying hospitals" to carry wounded from the field of battle and administer first aid, Wiesenthal then established two "horse stable hospitals" as he called them for prolonged treatment beyond the lines. One was in Baltimore. Somehow understanding that fetid bedding and stagnant water were linked with the transmission of disease, Wiesenthal ordered that all patients receive fresh straw bedding upon arrival.

At the first meeting of the Medical Society of Baltimore, which was held on December 15, 1788 at Stark's Tavern, Dr. Elisha Hall spoke on the necessity for regulations on the practice of "physic," and sketched a plan for a state medical society. Dr. Hall's plan, as it included all the precepts of the original 1799 charter of the Medical and Chirurgical Faculty of Maryland may well have been its foundation. Dr. Hall deferentially opened his address to his colleagues in the new Baltimore City society:

> "I offer a small sketch of a law which accompanies this address, for future regulation of the practice of Physic in this State...nothing but a heartfelt desire to promote the Public Good, our present and future deliberations, would have induced me to have acted...on the present

occasion...Several of our sister States have passed laws of this nature, and receive manifest benefit therefrom. The State of New York, the State of New Jersey, and Delaware, act as worthy examples, and their citizens now enjoy all those heartfelt sensations that arise from a conscious security in the integrity and professional abilities of their Family Physicians."

Wiesenthal's group disbanded after his death one year later, and before the establishment of a statewide organization. He was succeeded in his practice by his son, Andrew, whose unsuccessful attempt to found a proper medical college left him to continue his father's regimen of lectures from the Gay Street house. He received his marching orders from his father: "To rescue the Dignity of Physic from the horrid State into which it has plunged within these few Years and most especially since my Sickness will require a herculean effort...It will fall on your shoulders." With that in mind, Andrew Wiesenthal undertook the resurrection of the local Society, and added six physicians to the original group. In 1790, there were 13,524 citizens in Baltimore, with 30 physicians serving their medical needs.

The second group was also short-lived, for by June, 1790 the Society was engaged in a debate about the causes for its failure, and the last extant notes were taken on July 26th. A full page advertisement appeared on that date in the *Maryland Journal and Baltimore Daily Advertiser* taken out by a member of the Society who signed himself "A Spectator." It was in response to shadowy charges made by another Baltimore physician on June 21, 1790: "...We are open to reproach which some one may step in and cast upon us," Dr. George Buchanan wrote without naming who the "some one" may be. "...Some amongst us have stepped forward, with industry, to establish Societies, but others, of more intrigue, have succeeded in dissolving them, to the no small injury of themselves and the public..."

There were 17 physicians on the active roll of the Medical Society of Baltimore in 1790, and nine of them, if the advertisement headed "TO THE PUBLIC"can be believed, voted to dissolve their union. Nine was not a quorum according to the By-Laws and the author, who signed himself "Spectator," indicated that, perhaps by virtue of their combativeness, the nine prevailed in spite of that. He advises the nine to "retire from the theatre so ill suited to their genius and hide their blushes from a condemning world."

THE BALTIMORE CITY MEDICAL SOCIETY - A History

Others joined in bemoaning the failure of the Medical Society of Baltimore. One complained that:

> "The most zealous Members of the Society - those who alone could reflect credit upon the Institution - and upon whose Talents depended for its Existence and Support, finding after a mortifying experiment of several Months, that vexatious obstacles were perpetually raised against its Progress, and that the Object for which the Society was established was forgotten in the pitiful Quibbling which some delighted in, thought necessary to propose the dissolution...
>
> A Member of the late Medical Society
> June 24, 1790"

Some members of the original society did, however, continue to work toward a more orderly assembly of physicians, and to advocate for improved professional education and licensing. Drs. George Buchanan and George Brown of Baltimore, both of whom were close colleagues of the Drs. Weisenthal, were among the leaders who petitioned the Maryland legislature to establish a statewide organization. On January 20, 1799, the act which created the Medical and Chirurgical Faculty of the State of Maryland was passed in Annapolis. Baltimore City sent nine delegates to the organizational meetings. A Board of Governors was established, with seven members from the western shore and five from the Eastern Shore, and charged with the responsibility of licensing physicians either by testing their competency or examining their diplomas from credible medical colleges. The fine for practicing medicine without a license was set at $50.00 per incident.

Maryland's statewide Faculty was the sixth in the young nation. Its meetings have continued unabated since 1799, even during the difficult years of the Civil War. Throughout its history it has been supportive of local affiliates in Baltimore City and the counties, offering meeting space, organizational help and reorganization, tolerating some of the local societies' comings and goings and freely participating in efforts to spread information. During the 1870's, the Faculty rented meeting space to no fewer than three Baltimore societies at the same time. Officers of local societies have become officers of the Medical and Chirurgical Faculty.

Records of other organizations in the first half of the nineteenth century are scarce. A group called the "Medical Society of Baltimore" was begun in 1804, its first president being a Dr.

Dunkle, its secretary Dr. Davidge (presumably the namesake of the first building of the College of Medicine in Maryland, opened in 1812). The *Medical and Physical Recorder* of 1809 mentioned an 1807 group, the "Medical Association of Baltimore." Except for a single meeting at which a Dr. G. Williamson related the case of an 8-year old girl with metastasis (The patient was also taken with pleurisy and a severe inflammation of the brain. She survived those indignities, but in the process developed a violent dysentery and died) nothing else is known of the organization.

A "Society for the Promotion of Vaccination" was formed by Rev. Dr. Boyd, Bishop Carroll, and a William Gwynn in 1810. Dr. James Smith had established by 1802 the "Vaccine Institute" at his home on Calvert Street, where he provided free vaccination against yellow fever and smallpox. None of the three founders of the 1810 group was a doctor, but perhaps they were successful as promoters because *Niles' Weekly Register*, a national business newspaper published in Baltimore, reported in 1812 that it was common for the upper class in Baltimore to be vaccinated against smallpox, and to have their servants and slaves vaccinated as well.

Taneyhill's aforementioned 1881 address reported his having found in *The Medical and Surgical Journal* of April, 1840 a memorial that marked the passing of Dr. William Donaldson of Baltimore and noted that he was President of the "Medical Society of Baltimore" from 1822 through 1823. This was probably the same Society which was credited for the outline of a new Baltimore City Board of Health, voted upon by the City Council on June 28, 1820, and perhaps the same group founded by Drs. Dunkle and Davidge in 1804. . Dr. Donaldson was also one of the founders of the "Beneficial Society for the Prevention of Hydrophobia" in 1814, in concert with, among others, Dr. Samuel Baker.

This same *Journal* mentioned the "Baltimore Medical Society," with Dr. Samuel Baker as president from 1824 until 1826. Dr. Taneyhill did not say that this was the same organization as the Dunkle-Davidge-Donaldson group, and his chronicle is otherwise precise in its detail. As there were many competing groups, with confusingly-similar names, and since some folded following the passing of an important leader, any conclusion is guesswork. The local newspapers of the day often used different names for a single organization in the same article, complicating even further the task of distinguishing the early professional medical organizations in Baltimore. The only evidence that the organization endured beyond 1823 is a discussion in 1832 regarding the possible merger between the Medical Society of Baltimore and the Medico-Chirurgical Society of Baltimore (*not* the Medical and Chirurgical Faculty of Maryland; this was a Baltimore City organization).

In any case, nothing else is known for sure about this particular Medical Society of Baltimore, but its importance is established merely by the name of this president, for Samuel Baker was an important contributor to local medical organizations for more than a decade. Dr. Baker was a prominent Baltimore physician, holding a baccalaureate degree in the classics from Washington College in Chestertown, Maryland, and a medical degree from the University of Pennsylvania. In addition to his responsibilities as presiding officer of two organizations, Baker held the Chair of Malarial Medicine at the College of Medicine in Maryland and was an attending physician at the Baltimore Almshouse, the Baltimore General Dispensary and the Female Orphan Asylum. For several years he was the Chairman of the Medical and Chirurgical Faculty of Maryland Library Committee, and is credited with assembling the Faculty's first collection of books and manuscripts in 1830.

Dr. Baker was also the president of the Medico-Chirurgical Society of Baltimore, and in that capacity had a hand in drawing up one of the first "Codes of Medical Ethics" in the nation. Based largely on another Code of Medical Ethics, written in 1803 by Thomas Percival, M.D. for the doctors at Manchester Hospital in England, these formed the basis for the general code of the American Medical Association. The Medico-Chirurgical Society was begun in 1832, and the name Samuel Baker was among the three founders. Like earlier attempts to organize, the three physicians, Nathan R. Smith and J.H. Miller joining Dr. Baker, asked "How shall harmony of sentiment be established, and the dignity of the profession thus secured, but by frequent and frank intercourse? And how shall this be effected but by our systematic association?"

Probably because of Dr. Baker's involvement with the state organization's library, the sporadic Minutes of the Medico-Chirurgical Society of Baltimore from 1832 until 1838 survive. The first meeting established a constitution with a typically flowery, but significant, preamble:

> "The members of a liberal and enlightened Profession are in nothing so strongly contrasted with the empirical adventures as in their community of knowledge, of interests, and honor. The character of the medical Profession is elevated precisely in proportion to the freedom with which

information is reciprocally imparted, and to the common interest which is felt in the prosperity and reputation of the fraternity."

The Minutes, being the earliest extant such documents, reveal the workings of a Baltimore-based society and describe, by the Order of Business, an assembly that is first and foremost an instrument for finding cures. The group met semi-monthly. Each meeting began with the customary officers' reports and the presentation of candidates for admission. Following was a lecture, on topics such as "Asian Cholera - Contagious or Non-Contagious?" or "Does Neuralgia Depend Upon the Inflamation of Nervous Tissues?". Those present then engaged in debate about the lecture, and the meeting was closed by the relating of current cases which either baffled the physician or which were met with particular success. It is easy to imagine that this "talking shop" part of the agenda, not unlike modern rounds except for the physical absence of a patient, kept the members talking until late into the night.

In early 1833 the topic of a published fee table arose, and after several meetings during which the group labored over every line, a table was adopted. The Minutes document discussions regarding the fees themselves, but unfortunately are of little use without having the actual table at hand. No copies of the actual table exist, but the alterations made to the first draft indicate that the fee for "Cases of Gonorrhea and Syphilis (fee in advance)" was $50.00. "Tying large arteries in the case of wounds" had the same price tag. "First Consultation or Visit" cost $5.00.

There are no Medico-Chirurgical Society Minutes from October, 1835 until March, 1837, and abruptly in 1838 the minute book ends. Achieving a quorum for any meetings in 1837 and 1838 appeared all but impossible. There is no reason given, and no indication as to whether meetings continued beyond 1838. Dr. Baker passed away in 1835. In 1976, writing for the *Baltimore City Medical Society Newsletter*, President Richard L. London, M.D. stated that the Medico-Chirurgical Society survived, and assumed the role of medical education monitor for Baltimore following a proposal to establish such by the state Medical and Chirurgical Faculty. Dr. London went on to say that this same organization "re-organized into the Medical and Surgical Society of Baltimore" in 1855. Dr. London's statement is not footnoted.

Records of the state Faculty recalled "the Medico-Chirurgical Society which was already in former time a successful operation in

Baltimore, and whose meetings were for several years objects of much interest to the profession," and urged its revival. In any case, a new group was born, and maintained a relationship with the state group. Perhaps Dr. Baker's organization had continued after all.

Five members of this precursor to the Medical and Surgical Society of Baltimore were among the attendees at the first Annual Meeting of the American Medical Association, in Baltimore in May, 1848. Dr. John L. Yeates was among them. Dr. Yeates was born in Harford County and educated at the University of Maryland, where he received his degree in1822. His career crossed from the medical community to the political, as he served on the Baltimore City Council as well as on the Baltimore City School Commission. These experiences prepared him for one term as president of the Maryland Medical and Chirurgical Faculty, following which, in 1855, he presided for a single year over the Medical and Surgical Society of Baltimore. No records remain from the city group.

A vast array of other short-lived assemblies dots the pre-Civil War medical landscape of Baltimore, some remembered only because of a single line in a Baltimore City Directory or in the biography of a notable Baltimore physician. For example, in 1853 the "Baltimore Pathological Society" held its first meeting. Among its founders are several prominent Baltimore doctors: Dr. D. Steuart, Dr. Pottenger, and Dr. Charles Frick. Of this organization nothing else was recorded until 1872, when according to Dr. John R. Quinan, in his magnum opus *Medical Annals of Baltimore*, it folded after the conviction of one of its members for medical misconduct.

Each of these small organizations seemed to suffer from the same malady: They were unable to sustain the long-term interest of local physicians, and thus unable to collect enough dues to stay afloat. As late as December, 1878, in the Baltimore Medical Association, the most successful of the pre-1900 societies, Treasurer Dr. Judson Gilman complained that "...only 32 of 89 members have paid their dues this year, and money is needed to pay the rent. I hope those present who have not paid will do so tonight." Mergers between competing associations were often considered simply to boost membership and attendance at meetings.

Between 1859 and 1866 there were apparently no organized local medical associations in Baltimore. The Maryland Medical and Chirurgical Faculty reported indifferent attendance at its irregular meetings. Eventually the only meeting was held annually to elect new officers and pay the bills, barely keeping the state Faculty alive.

There was no local medical society active until after the war. For most of the Civil War years the city was under the aforementioned cannon of General Benjamin Butler, who ruled Baltimore under martial law. Organizations and clubs either run by southern sympathizers or suspected of rebel bias were banned and public meetings were forbidden. Many leading citizens, including Mayor George William Brown, the Baltimore City Police Commissioner, a former Maryland Governor and a host of state delegates and newspaper editors were imprisoned for all or parts of the war, many at Fort McHenry.

"The profession to which we belong, once venerated on account of its antiquity - its various and profound science - its elegant literature - its polite accomplishments - its virtues - has become corrupt and degenerate to the forfeiture of its social position and, with it, of the homage it formerly received spontaneously and universally."

With those words, Nathan Chapman, M.D, opened the first annual session of the American Medical Association in Baltimore in 1848. The spirit behind the new national organization was a young physician, Dr. Nathan S. Davis, who at age 29 conceived the idea of an association to lift the profession of physic to the dignified level in American society where it once was and still belonged. Dr. Davis, in concert with 80 representatives from medical societies and colleges in 16 states, had drawn up four proposals in May, 1846, which sought to develop uniform standards for the conferring of the degree of Medical Doctor, assure that young men entering the profession had the suitable formal training, and bind each practitioner to a national code of medical ethics. The American Medical Association was formally founded in May, 1847.

The first state society, launched in New Jersey in 1766, was followed by a society in Maryland in 1799 (the Medical and Chirurgical Faculty, which is still in existence and is among the few societies to retain the old English nomenclature). A dozen more flourished by the time Dr. Davis, a delegate to the New York State Medical Society, drew up his manifesto for a uniquely American association. *The New England Journal of Medicine* published its first issue in 1820. Ether had been in use as an anesthesia for only one year.

The AMA was organized as a collective of state, county and local medical societies and medical schools. Dues were set at $3.00/year and delegates were urged to return home and establish local affiliates.

In declaring war on quackery and the proliferation of snake oil home remedies, the Association set a mission which it was hoped would elevate both medicine and those who practiced it. Ethics, in addition to medical education of both the public and physicians and the advancement of science dominated the agenda of the AMA until the Civil War. In 1849, the Committee on Medical Education studied the curricula of medical universities in Europe and compared them to those in the United States, with an eye toward the regularization of medical training. That same year, the association published a resolution encouraging members to "enlighten the public mind in regards to the duties and the responsibilities of the medical profession and their just claims to the confidence of the public." In 1842 the AMA pilloried the conditions suffered by European immigrants, who crossed the ocean in the abysmal conditions of the steerage class, thus beginning a long and diligent effort to address public health issues.

Over 150 years later, the AMA continues its mission of making Americans more intelligent consumers of health care, of training practitioners to deliver the finest care in the world, of holding those caregivers to a rigid standard of ethics and of demanding that our elected officials guarantee the highest level of public health.

The Baltimore Medical Association

Thus it was with the recent memory of practicing medicine either on the battlefield or in a city under siege that the Baltimore Medical Association came to be in 1866. Minutes from meetings from 1869 through the period leading up to the 1904 reorganization which established the modern Baltimore City Medical Society tell the story of an organization that alternately struggled and prospered in its nearly four decades.

Beginning with the very first meeting, at the Maryland Medical and Chirurgical Faculty office at 47 Calvert Street, the Association welded a close and beneficial relationship with the statewide organization. In October, 1869, when the state group abandoned Calvert Street for its new home at 60 Courtland Street, the Baltimore Medical Association followed. Both organizations would be more comfortable than in the old "two-story-and-an-attic" rowhouse on Calvert near Baltimore Street, where they shared rooms on the second floor and presumably the attic space beneath the sloping roof. On the ground floor was the headquarters of the state Faculty. The front room of the second floor was a meeting room used by the Association and other groups, and the library was in the rear of the same floor.

The Calvert Street house was typical of thousands of other 1815-1830 Federal style rowhouses in Baltimore, with red bricks laid in flemish bond (an alternating pattern of ends and sides of brick, neatly laid with thin, uniform mortar joints) and a shingled roof, gently sloping toward the street. The roof, penetrated by one gable, was by 1869 clad in seamed rows of tin, but the original wooden shingles were probably still in place beneath the metal. Access to the meeting rooms was doubtless through the first floor front room, and up a narrow, tightly-wound, walled spiral staircase which would have been a challenge for the claustrophobic. The house's original source of heat would have been four fireplaces, and as Baltimore was slow to adopt the cast iron stoves that graced old hearths in other east coast cities, it is likely that the open fireplace still dominated one wall of the physicians' meeting rooms. As early as 1855, Dr. John L. Yeates's Medical and Surgical Society of Baltimore, paid the Faculty $175.00 in annual rent to use the Calvert Street rooms for its semi-monthly meetings.

It is difficult to imagine a less suitable venue for serious medical discussions. The members of the Baltimore Medical Association would have huddled beneath low ceilings in their cramped space, those near the fire baking in the winter and those distant from it (the rooms were nearly 25 feet wide) shivering. During the summer the second floor would have been a steamy oven, the several vents cut through the roof at its peak providing little in the way of ventilation.

More appropriate rooms were located at number 60 Courtland Street, and in September of 1869 the state Faculty purchased the building for $5,700.00. The Baltimore Medical Association participated in the formal opening of the building, which must have been a grand affair as it occupied two full days, October 28th and 29th. The Association continued its bi-weekly meetings, but remained on Courtland Street initially only for one year, moving its operations to the Chatard Building in 1870. The doctors met briefly at the home of President John R. Uhler on Greene Street, and in 1874 rented space above the Methodist Book Concern for $100.00/year. Finally, in 1877 the Association rented space again from the state Faculty at its new home on Fayette Street between Liberty and Howard Streets, where they stayed for many years.

Throughout the moves, the Association continued its agenda of medical education, but spent increasing amounts of time addressing issues of public health and lobbying the new City Hall for improvements in the health prospects for all Baltimoreans. In April of 1872 the Association discussed and approved a resolution calling for the establishment of a special hospital near Baltimore for contagious and infectious disease. The members determined that a portion of the beds should be appropriated to paying patients and a portion allocated to non-paying patients. Later that same year, in partnership with a sister organization, the Medical and Surgical Society of Baltimore, the Association appointed a committee to study relations between physicians and druggists.

An ongoing issue for general practitioners in the late nineteenth century was the role of the specialist. It was at first considered a problem more of ethics than of practical medicine, for the contention was that specialists demeaned the role of the family doctor and strove to steal his patients. There were discussions that would have led to the barring of members from consulting with specialists at all, and in 1873 the Association compromised by adopting a resolution of the Baltimore Pathological Society. Specialists were admonished to follow the same Code of Ethics as that used by the Association, which banned public advertising. The agreement forbade general practitioners who were members of either organization from consulting with specialists who violated the rules. The matter of generalist vs. specialist was not resolved for decades, but this resolution provided at least a peace treaty.

Besides the larger issues of ethics and professional relationships, a vital dialogue was maintained that addressed the average practice on a more nuts-and-bolts basis. Discussions from 1874 through 1876 addressed syphilis (inspired by the case of a syphilitic man whose healthy wife had given birth to a child born "a pale, shrunken, mummified-looking object") migraines, ancestral intelligence and heredity, the relationship between the offensive odors of the Basin (now the Inner Harbor) and disease, and yellow fever. The odd specimen was also presented, or the very odd specimen in the case of the "kitten, born dead, having one head and two bodies" that Dr. Ellis brought to the November 13, 1882 meeting.

At the November 18, 1869 meeting, Dr. Williams mentioned that he had used chloroform to control hysteria, but that his patients afterwards suffered from uncontrollable vomiting. As late as May, 1872, Dr. Morris admitted to still using bleeding to control sunstroke, but that he lost many patients anyway. It was suggested that ice was a more reliable remedy. On December 10, 1878, Dr. J.H. Smith "read a long and interesting paper on 'Allopathy and Homeopathy' and predicted the downfall of homeopathy while regular medicine would continue to flourish."

Two partnerships have been mentioned, one between the Baltimore Medical Association and Baltimore Pathological Society, which was created in 1853 and was near its last days when it joined with the Association to address the specialist dilemma. The other was with the Medical and Surgical Society of Baltimore, which opened its doors in February, 1871, as the "East Baltimore Medical Society."

Ostensibly, the creation of a new east Baltimore organization was so that physicians living and practicing in Old Town, Fells Point, and other neighborhoods would have a place to meet closer to home. The new group was modeled after the Baltimore Medical Association, for its first set of by-laws (now part of the Baltimore City Medical Society archives) is a pencil-amended copy of the Association's own 1866 Constitution and By-Laws.

The east Baltimore group adopted the Association's Order of Business, with minor alterations. In addition to presentations on subjects of particular medical interest, the founders considered it important to include discussions on general scientific topics. Just before each Adjournment, the original By-Laws calls for "Humourous Discussions," but that line is struck out in pencil, as perhaps the founders decided that a little levity was inappropriate.

Beginning with an ambitious weekly schedule, the Medical and Surgical Society of Baltimore, as the east Baltimore group called itself formally, selected meeting places "east of Central Av. South of Orleans St. West of Wolfe Street & North of Canton Av." in the heart of east Baltimore. Like the Baltimore Medical Association, the east Baltimore group elected officers annually. Unlike that group, they established two permanent committees: The Committee of Lectures and Discussions and the Committee of Medical Literature. The former was to choose topics for presentation on a weekly basis, announcing the new topic at the prior week's meeting. The literature committee was mandated to "present to the Society, at the last meeting of each month, an Abstract of all interesting papers that may be contained in the journals published during that month."

In the archives of the modern Baltimore City Medical Society, the original Constitution and By-Laws of the physicians from east Baltimore are recorded in a small volume, its pages yellowed and fragile from over a century of life. On the inside front cover, beneath the seal of the Library of the Medical and Chirurgical Faculty of Maryland, is the note that this slim pamphlet was presented by Dr. A.F. Erich. Augustus F. Erich made his first appearance in a Baltimore City Directory in 1863, when he was listed as practicing medicine at 114 South Broadway.

Before his death in 1886, Dr. Erich, whose speciality was gynecology, compiled an impressive professional dossier, including positions of leadership in several organizations. In addition to being a Founder and first President of the Medical and Surgical Society of

Baltimore, he was a member of the Baltimore Medical Association. At the October 23, 1882 meeting of the Association, he led a discussion about several very virulent cases of diphtheria he observed in a single household.

Dr. Erich attended meetings of the Baltimore Medical Association on a regular basis in the early 1880's, and as the Minutes report, regularly either led or participated in discussions on a variety of topics from "What Should We Do With Chloroform?" to "Treatment of Uterine Hemorrhage." He served on the Association's Executive Committee in 1882, but beginning in the spring of 1883 his name no longer appeared with the attending members. In 1885 he again presided over the organization that he founded, the Medical and Surgical Society of Baltimore.

Erich is worthy of special consideration in the history of local medical organizations, because not only did he organize one and become an active member of others, he also edited *Baltimore Physician and Surgeon* and taught chemistry and gynecology at the College of Physicians and Surgeons. In 1877 he founded Women's Hospital, where he remained the surgeon-in-chief until his death. His daughter, Louise Erich, was graduated from the Woman's Medical College in Baltimore in 1895 and her practice developed with a specialty in orthopaedics as it related to women's health.

While the Baltimore Medical Association met on the second and fourth Monday of every month, in the state Medical and Chirurgical Faculty offices (moving to St. Paul and Saratoga Streets in 1886 in concert with the state Faculty), the east Baltimore physicians continued to meet weekly at their hall at Baltimore and Eden Street, just north of Fells Point. In 1896, they finally moved into the Medical and Chirurgical Faculty headquarters, then at 847 North Eutaw Street. This move brought a number of state and local organizations under the same roof: The Baltimore Medical Association, the Medical and Surgical Society of Baltimore, the Baltimore Academy of Medicine, the Gynecological and Obstetric Society of Baltimore, the Clinical Society of Maryland, and the Maryland Medical and Chirurgical Faculty.

In 1873, membership at Baltimore Medical Association meetings had declined so dramatically that the President reported an inability to pay the bills. Perhaps because of dwindling interest, as early as 1876, Dr. Isaac Edmonson Atkinson suggested at a Baltimore Medical Association meeting that there were benefits to be derived from "a union of all the Societies in the City," and moved to form a committee to study such a merger. The committee reported the following October that such a coalition was impractical and the matter was dropped.

But the idea must have seemed more realistic when it arose in 1897 and every group was holding its meetings in the same building. On October 25th of that year, Dr. David Streett bemoaned that the regular meetings of the Baltimore Medical Association were sparsely attended, and that perhaps a merger might boost the audience and lift the organization into greater prominence in the medical community. Dr. C. Urban Smith argued that all it may take to attract more members was the addition of a social hour at the end of every meeting. Dr. Streett disagreed. "What we want is more papers," he is quoted in the evening's Minutes, and a way to accomplish that would be a merger with the Medical and Surgical Society of Baltimore. Dr. John I. Pennington suggested that each society could, after the merger, maintain some of its sovereignty by becoming a Section of the state Faculty. As with other issues like this one, a committee was formed to investigate.

One month later, Dr. John D. Blake reported to the Baltimore Medical Association that the Medical and Surgical Society would be amenable to a union as long as the name was the Baltimore Medical and Surgical Association. They also wished to keep their accustomed Thursday meeting nights. By December of 1897 the decision to combine was made, and at a joint meeting of the Baltimore Medical Association and the Medical and Surgical Society of Baltimore arrangements for the consolidation were completed. Following a preliminary meeting of the new organization, Dr. John Schwatka was chosen as President and Dr. Charles T. Harper secretary. Dr. G. Lane Taneyhill then moved that the first year of the Baltimore Medical and Surgical Association begin on January 1, 1898 and that the Trustees of the Medical and Chirurgical Faculty be advised that the relationship with the two separate groups be dissolved in favor of the new one.

As it turns out, the meeting nights were changed in 1898 to the second and fourth Friday of every month. Minutes from the period immediately following the union and the eventual reorganization in 1904, when the modern Baltimore City Medical Society was created, are lost. Presumably the regular Order of Business of committee reports, medical presentations and case studies continued. Many of the same faces that met together for the first time in January, 1898 were around the table when the Baltimore City Medical Society emerged in 1904: Taneyhill, Atkinson, Neff, Blake, and Friedenwald among others. Dr. John Neff could recall the meeting in Dr. Gerald E. Morgan's office on February 26, 1866. A new name on the roster in the closing days of the nineteenth century was that of Eugene Fauntleroy Cordell, M.D. Dr. Cordell became the unofficial historian and the first century of medical associations in the city of Baltimore came to an end with his 1903 observations:

"And what a great period that was for progress and research - the nineteenth century - which we would fain believe to be the greatest of them all!...The specialties all come to the front. Clinical teaching and work are conspicuous. More exact methods and instrumental aids of all sorts are introduced. All the sciences are called on to contribute. Ausculation and percussion, improved microscopes, the ophthalmoscope, laryngoscope, endoscope and specula of various sorts...Pathology and histology are cultivated with increasing success...With the discovery of anesthesia surgery takes a great bound forward."

"The purpose of this society shall be to bring into one organization the physicians of Baltimore City, so that by the frequent interchange of views and unity of action, they may best promote the advance of medical science, elevate professional standards and improve public health conditions; and, with the County Societies, to form the Medical and Chirurgical Faculty of Maryland, and through it, with the other State associations, to form and maintain the American Medical Association."

-The Baltimore City Medical Society
Preamble to the Constitution and By-Laws
April 15, 1904

"The Name and Title of this Organization Shall be the 'Baltimore City Medical Society'."

The Medical Profession in Baltimore Enters the 20th Century

In a clear and eminently legible hand, Dr. John Ruhrah carefully recorded the proceedings of the founding committee on the numbered and ruled pages of a book now neatly bound in burgundy, with gilt letters on its bound edge announcing that inside are contained the Minutes of the Baltimore City Medical Society from April, 1904 through November, 1915. The black ink has faded to charcoal, but Dr. Ruhrah's precise penmanship appropriately dignifies the occasion to all who have read it since.

Among the physicians who made and seconded motions, who served on a Nominating Committee and who before the close of the April 15, 1904 meeting accepted positions of responsibility, were the city's most prominent practitioners. Dr. Harry Friedenwald, the new society's first President, was a turn-of-the-century renaissance man. A lecturer at the University of Maryland in diseases of the eye and ear, he was also an important figure in the international Zionist movement. Dr. Friedenwald boasted the most important collection of ancient manuscripts of Jewish medical history in the world which in 1930 he left to the University of Palestine.

Dr. Henry Ottrage Reik, the Chairman of the Committee on Reorganization, was a well known eye and ear surgeon who would go on to write three landmark books about ENT treatment and surgery. Dr. William Sidney Thayer was the successor to Dr. William Osler at Johns Hopkins and by 1904 had already written one important book about malarial fever in Baltimore and several important articles for journals. Dr. Thayer went on to become president of the AMA in 1928, and was so well known internationally that when Queen Elizabeth and King Albert of the Belgian royal family visited the United States, he was their host in Baltimore. While at the Mental Health Clinic at Hopkins, he introduced the royal visitors to a well-known psychiatrist who happened to be on duty. "May I present the Queen of Rumania," Thayer recalled having said. The psychiatrist responded "And how long has the lady believed herself to be Queen of the Rumanians?"

Royal visits aside, Baltimore City was, as the twentieth century opened, firmly the center of medical thought and practice in Maryland and, to a large extent, throughout the nation and the world. The University of Maryland School of Medicine was founded in 1807. Johns Hopkins University was founded in 1874 and the hospital opened in 1889. The medical school followed in 1893 and immediately became a model for schools across the country. Dr. William Osler, the first Physician-in-Chief at Hopkins, once joked with Dr. William Welch, its first dean of the medical school, "Welch, we were lucky to get in as professors, for I am sure that neither you nor I could ever get in as students."

Dr. John Beale Davidge was in 1904 already an historical icon among physicians whose practices were on different continents from the hall that bears his name at the University of Maryland. Over a century had passed since he admitted the first of his many students to his private Anatomical Hall in 1800. The university that honors him became a part of the University of Maryland in 1812. It was one of many pioneering efforts that by 1904 had rightfully put Baltimore on the medical map: The first American lectures on dentistry were delivered at the University of Maryland, and the first American dental college was established here in 1840. The School of Pharmacy was the first of its kind in the American South. Dr. Harvey Cushing, the father of modern neurosurgery, had been the first to use x-ray diagnosis in an operating room in Baltimore. The University of Maryland's Dr. William Frick wrote the first American textbook on ophthalmology. The first surgeon to don rubber gloves in an operating room anywhere in the world was Dr. William Halsted, at Johns Hopkins. So as the physicians worked to create the Baltimore City Medical Society, they were in reality building one of the most important local associations of medical professionals in the nation.

That the doctors meeting at the state Faculty in 1904 considered themselves a "Committee on Reorganization" confirms that there was still a local society functioning in 1904. The Medical and Surgical Association indeed had a listing in the Baltimore City Directories from the time of the 1897 merger until 1905, publishing the names of their officers and the fact that the group met twice monthly at the state Faculty headquarters on Eutaw Street.

The reorganizations were a small part of a national plan of the American Medical Association in Chicago and affected the smallest local component societies in every state. By 1900, the AMA boasted that 9,000 of an estimated 100,000 physicians in the United States were members, and that 15,000 physicians regularly read the *Journal of the American Medical Association*. A more organized structure was necessary to accommodate the growth and meet the expanding mission of the AMA. As the twentieth century dawned, the AMA held its Annual Meeting in Atlantic City, New Jersey. One of the most important proposals to emerge from the meeting was the establishment of a Committee on Organization to study the current alignment of the local and state groups with the national association and to recommend changes.

Substantial amendments to the AMA constitution were ready for consideration at the 1901 Annual Meeting. A new House of Delegates was to be made up of representatives from each state medical society, composed of one delegate for every 500 members in the state. Any approved member of a local group that operated within a state assembly was granted membership in the AMA after making application, proving his or her good standing in the medical community and paying the annual dues.

State societies and faculties were ordered to reorganize along those same lines, and where no local society existed the AMA strongly urged the state organization to establish one. A return to a more scientific focus was mandated for those societies which, like the Baltimore group, had deleted scientific Sections from their agendas. Attention to legislative matters took a new and higher priority. Thus in 1904, when Baltimore doctors gathered, it was "In pursuance of a call issued by the Special Committee on Reorganization of the Medical and Chirurgical Faculty of Maryland, and authorized by the Executive Committee thereof."

Reorganization Under AMA Guidelines

To say that the new Baltimore City Medical Society was radically different from its forebears would be an exaggeration, but the organization outlined in the 1904 Constitution is notably different in several ways. Following the tack of the AMA, which established its first Committee on National Legislation in 1901, the Baltimore City Medical Society created a Committee on Public Health and Legislation. This was the first official acknowledgment that a local Baltimore medical society should serve as an advocate for improving sanitation and public health through lobbying. It also marked a period when government was becoming more active in health issues. What the AMA was doing in Washington the Baltimore City Medical Society was to do on Holliday Street, under the golden dome of City Hall.

Consisting of three members to be appointed annually by the president, the new committee was charged with the responsibility of not only helping to enact sanitary and medical laws, but of enforcement of those laws as well. Working closely with the Committee on Public Policy and Legislation of the state Faculty, both bodies would contribute to the finding and prosecuting of "pretenders in this City." The role of the Public Health and

Legislation Committee grew rapidly, so much so that by the December 5, 1905 meeting it was proposed that an auxiliary legislative committee was needed simply to address the matters of medical law and lawmaking. An auxiliary committee of ten members was nominated by President W.S. Thayer, M.D.

A Committee for Programs and Scientific Work was established, to consist of the President, the Vice President and the Secretary. It was the duty of this committee to "promote the scientific and social functions of the Society by arranging attractive programs for each meeting." Moribund since the 1890's, the idea of technical Sections was resuscitated in the 1904 Constitution, and the Society delineated five specialties which should be addressed by individual Section committees: 1) Clinical medicine, pathology and surgery, 2) Obstetrics and gynecology, 3) Neurology and psychiatry, 4) Ophthalmology and otology, and 5) Laryngology and rhinology.

Gone from the Order of Business are the familiar case studies that were a staple of earlier groups. There are short technical talks, such as the paper read by Dr. H. Warren Buckler on the use of nitrous oxide as an anaesthetic in December, 1907. Much more time at the now only twice-a-year meetings is devoted to Society business, the admission of new members, and, increasingly, the larger issues of medical ethics and public health.

Along those lines, the new Baltimore City Medical Society hit the ground running. At the same meeting at which an Auxiliary Legislative Committee was approved the first proclamation regarding a public health issue was also unanimously accepted: "Whereas the production of black smoke in the city of Baltimore especially by locomotives is a nuisance injuriously affecting human health and the comfort of a large part of the residence portion of the city and whereas it is an unnecessary nuisance, and is already partially prohibited by law...be it resolved that the Medical Society of Baltimore City [sic.] regards with satisfaction the movement now being inaugurated by certain public spirited citizens of Baltimore to suppress this nuisance..."

Just a month later, at a special meeting called for February 2, 1906, the problem of patent, or proprietary, medicines was discussed. Earlier organizations had always advocated strongly against the very existence of these medicines. Just forty years earlier, when the Baltimore Medical Association was formed, among the activities that could result in a physician's rejection were "Giving a certificate of the efficacy of any secret medicine...Receiving a percentage or any other remuneration from druggists on prescriptions, or being in any manner interested in the sale of drugs and medicines." In 1899, the new editor of the *Journal of the American Medical Association*, Dr. George H. Simmons, had begun an unrelenting campaign against patent medicines in all forms. The Baltimore City Medical Society's campaign bears a thorough telling, it being their first venture as activists into local politics.

Mr. Edward Bok, editor of *The Ladies Home Journal*, had written to the Society, seeking support for a Bill pending before the State legislature requiring that the contents of any proprietary medicine be printed on the label. Delegate Joseph E. Godwin, the chairman of the Baltimore City Delegation in Annapolis, spoke at the February, 1906 Society meeting in support of the Bill that he had introduced based on Bok's suggestions but altered to track Maryland law. "He advised early action," the meeting Minutes reported, "as the opposition has already become active." A committee of three was selected to speak for the Society in favor of the Bill, and the decision to support the Godwin Bill was passed unanimously.

What ensued was a hard-learned lesson in political reality. On April 5, 1906, the Special Committee on Patent Medicine and Legislation reported on the machinations of everyone involved in the ill-fated Bill. Society members visited every newspaper and every editor solemnly promised to report accurately on the debate. Those that did so, however, relegated the copy to the inner depths of their papers. One, the *Baltimore American and Commercial Daily Advertiser*, published a letter from A.C. Meyer, billed as a "special dispatch from a prominent druggist." Mr. Meyer condemned the proposed law, as might be expected of the proprietor of A.C. Meyer and Company, manufacturer of "Dr. Bull's Cough Syrup - For the Cure of Coughs and Colds" and "Salvation Oil - The Greatest Cure on Earth for Pain! It Stands Without Rival!".

The Society replied by calling a public meeting, sending out postcards announcing the meeting and urging citizens to support the Bill. Members visited churches, neighborhood improvement associations and civic clubs to advocate passage. The response that the Minutes noted in particular was of local pharmacists, who "were stirred most wonderfully, until they rose 'en masse', went to Annapolis one hundred strong, not to aid in the passage, but to use every method to defeat it, the whole trade with rare exceptions." Every Baltimore daily reported the druggists' campaign on the front page.

Undeterred, the Society called upon the Retail Druggists Association to form a committee so that the two organizations could pound out a compromise Bill of which everyone could approve. Such a meeting was scheduled, taking place on the train to Annapolis as both committees went to a meeting with Delegate Godwin. Compromise was reached, and Godwin withdrew his Bill, replacing it with one drawn by the physicians and pharmacists.

"This marvelous Remedy is beyond question one of the Greatest Medical Discoveries of the Century!"

During the two months in 1906 when the physicians of the Baltimore City Medical Society were visiting local newspaper editors, speaking to community organizations, churches and fraternal groups, and lobbying hard in Annapolis to have approved a Bill which would mandate that all patent medicines carried on their labels a list of their ingredients, the following exclamation-laden advertisements were among hundreds that appeared regularly in Baltimore newspapers:

"IF NURSING MOTHERS READ THIS THERE WILL BE FEWER LITTLE WHITE COFFINS
Mothers who take TAY-LOID LITHIA SELTZ while nursing their babies keep in perfect health and save the little ones from sickness and death...TAY-LOID LITHIA SELTZ (An Honest Non-Secret Home Remedy) is a springtime cleansing medicine for old and young alike which filters the blood, moves the bowels, makes a lazy liver work, and carries off waste, ferment and germs!
At M.S. Kahn's and all drug stores, 25¢"

"YOUR TONGUE IS COATED!
That's bad business, Bill! What were you eating? It doesn't matter because *it is your bowels that talk now, every time you open your mouth*...That doesn't help your popularity! *CASCARETS* are harmless, pleasant & convenient. Carry the ten cent box in your pocket!"

"DR. GREENE'S *NERVURA* has cured thousands and will cure you!
This marvelous remedy is beyond question one of the greatest medical discoveries of the century...If you are wise, if you desire to regain your health, you will be cured by DR. GREENE'S *NERVURA* Blood and Nerve Remedy. It is the essence of power, strength, energy and health!"

"At Home, CURE RHEUMATISM - *HANCOCK'S LIQUID SUPLHUR*
Nature's greatest germicide. Such a certain cure that we guarantee it to cure acne, eczema, dandruff, ringworm, prickly heat, diptheria, catarrh, cancer, sore throat, cuts and diseases of the scalp.

BOWEL POISON!
If your skin is disfigured by eruptions, humors, blotches. If your skin is scaly and rough. If you feel tired and worn out, your nerves weak, cross and depressed...If you have these DANGER SIGNALS they point unerringly to BOWEL POISON! Try **SMITH'S PINEAPPLE & BUTTERNUT PILLS!** *Nature's Laxative*

The creators of these miracle cures depended on tricking the public into believing that things from which everyone suffers from time to time - irritability, constipation, lethargy and tired muscles - were **DANGER SIGNALS!** All one had to do was to get one's bowels cleansed, blood filtered, liver de-acidified, and Dr. Whomever's Miracle Elixir was exactly the ticket.

They also handsomely padded the advertising coffers of newspapers and journals. So it was no wonder that the Baltimore City Medical Society's letters and articles to force these home nostrums off the shelf "of every drug store", or at least reveal the opiates and harsh diuretics and laxatives that they contained, ended up buried on page seven.

In the meantime, a petition circulated by the Emerson Drug Company (makers of Bromo Seltzer), A.C. Meyer and Company, and the Cafeeno Company, had gathered signatures of 300 Baltimore druggists in opposition. The compromise legislation failed. The Society responded with naive indignation. "You will doubtless recall the attack made upon the Medical Profession...Whether the fact that many local druggists hold stock in some of the headache concerns influenced them or not we are unable to say." The episode, however, concluded on a positive note: "...while the action has not resulted in a concrete legislation along this line, the issue was so vigorously presented, that it compelled the Patent Medicine People to aid in the passage of a Narcotics Law."

Ethics, Public Health and a Looming War

Increasing amounts of time were devoted to topics of medical ethics as the Baltimore City Medical Society grew. The ever-present question of the admission of practitioners who have any connection at all to homeopathy or "sectarian" medicine, became important as the society sought ways to boost paying membership. Homeopathy, the practice of treating a disease by administering minute doses of an agent that would in healthy persons result in symptoms of the same disease, was considered less than legitimate medicine. Though a homeopathic college existed in Baltimore, practitioners needed only to have studied on their own to hang out their shingles. The By-Laws were clear. Any physician who was legally qualified to practice medicine in Baltimore was eligible for membership, unless that applicant was "ostensibly practising homeopathy, or is affiliated with homeopathic colleges, hospitals or societies." The AMA was indecisive on the question, preferring to leave the decision to each state or local society.

A test case was proffered in the person of Dr. O. Edward Janney His name was on the list of potential new members at the December 4, 1906 Annual Meeting. Countless members spoke on his behalf:

"A most desirable member". Dr. Janney desired admission to the Medical Society, but refused to resign his membership from the Homeopathic Society. The Boston Medical Society had already opened the door to non-traditional practitioners, but Baltimore physicians were less willing to follow their example. "This question has exercised the Board very much," complained Board of Censors Chairman Dr. C.E. Brack.

Heated discussion followed, some members of the Board believing that it was time to recognize homeopathy, as long as the member met all the other requirements of the society. Others, like Dr. C. Urban Smith, argued that if homeopathy could be construed as "sectarian" medicine the decision was clear and Janney must be rejected. In the end they threw up their hands, and without first amending the By-Laws took a vote on the entire list of new members. Janney was, along with every other applicant, admitted. In one form or another, including the consideration of practitioners of chiropractic and acupuncture in more recent times, the issue would continue to vex the Society.

For years the presence of Dr. Janney and other homeopathic physicians, was quietly tolerated. In December, 1908, the Board acknowledged that among its members were two physicians who also served on the homeopathic examining board. One chose to resign. A "Don't ask, don't tell" non-policy was, without a vote, reluctantly acknowledged, and if an applicant had the required endorsement of two members that was all that was necessary for admittance. The Board of Censors repeated its intention of refusing applications from "known homeopaths," saying that "We desire to call the attention of the society to the need of new members, but wish at the same time to emphasize that no matter how greatly we need the influx of new members, the Board will not endorse practitioners who are not strictly eligible."

The question of physicians who legitimately practiced medicine while at the same time operating retail drug stores was equally difficult but more clear-cut. Nothing in the By-Laws barred these doctors, and it was the opinion of the Board of Censors that they were eligible for membership. The Board decided in 1907 to await a verdict of the entire membership. A year passed, and the 1908 amendments to the By-Laws minced no words in their decision: "Any physician who shall procure a patent for a remedy or a surgical instrument, or who sells or deals in patent medicines or nostrums, or who shall enter into an agreement with an apothecary...to receive pecuniary compensation for sending patients to that apothecary shall be disqualified from becoming or remaining a member." Ownership of shares of stock in a company manufacturing "secret" remedies was equally forbidden.

By-law amendments like this one occupied much of the agendas of Annual Meetings as the Baltimore City Medical Society solidified its role as an advocate for quality health care, improvements in public health and sanitation, and the elevation of the profession. The organization grew rapidly, from 37 members in 1904 to 611 as Europe went to war in 1914. Public health drew the Society closer to City Hall, and Mayor J. Barry Mahool addressed the Society in1908, asking its support for a "water loan" that would finance the expansion of the Loch Raven reservoir and bring clean water to Baltimore City. Two years later the Society found itself talking about whether the Jones Falls should be converted to a sewer.

Treatment afforded those suffering from alcoholism was criticized by the Society in 1911, pointing out that alcoholics were sent by the court to institutions promising rapid cures, one of which was owned by a practicing physician who had not passed the requirements of the State Board of Medical Examiners. The cures frequently failed, to the detriment of the Baltimore City treasury. The Society voted a resolution to condemn this practice, making no suggestions as to how it may be improved.

Meeting dates were sporadic in the period just before World War I. The original By-Laws did not specify the frequency or dates of meetings, and early practice was to meet but semi-annually. On October 17, 1913 it was proposed that the Society meet bi-weekly, on the first and third Fridays of each month, and the motion passed.

In April, 1914, the Society hosted a panel discussion about the medical profession and its coverage in the newspapers. Among the panel members was Henry Louis Mencken. Two years earlier someone from the Society had carefully compiled a report on local newspapers and found that "the names of thirty-one different doctors appeared in the morning paper during the month in connection with patients, or operations; in other words, purely medical matters..." This smacked of advertising, and a Committee was formed to investigate. The doctors were called before the Committee, and to a man they denied any responsibility for the publication of their names. From the 1914 meeting came a Resolution to work with local editors to arrive at a method of dealing with medical reports.

As World War I raged in France, the Baltimore City Medical Society turned its attention to the lessons learned under fire in Europe. Dr. J.A.C. Colston opened an October, 1915 seminar on battlefield conditions and military hospitals with a talk on "Personal Experiences at the Red Cross Hospital at Pau, France," and two other talks followed about conditions at an American Woman's Hospital in Devonshire, England and a Red Cross Hospital in Germany. As the sense that America would eventually enter the war grew, the Minutes became crowded with discussions and presentations on wartime medicine. The Baltimore City and County Medical Societies held a joint meeting in November, 1916 during which a series of films on French surgery at field hospitals was screened. Accounts of the horrendous slaughters at Verdun, Delville Wood and the Somme appeared in Baltimore newspapers and the meetings of the Society took an even more serious tone, so much so that on January 7, 1916, when "a professional contortionist and dislocationist requested the privilege of giving an exhibition before the Society" the proposal was tabled without discussion.

When the University of Maryland announced a course in "Military Medicine and Camp Sanitation," the Baltimore City Medical Society encouraged members to attend in March, 1917. The war became a frequent topic at the meetings until after the Armistice in November, 1918. Four days after the unarmed American merchantman Algonquin was sunk by a German U-boat, before the United States entered the war, the District of Columbia Medical Society was invited to attend a meeting addressing medical preparedness at Osler Hall, Johns Hopkins University. A week later, after it was learned that three other American ships had suffered the same fate, the Baltimore Society and the Maryland League for National Defense presented the film "The Army & Navy." Two weeks after that, on April 6, 1917, America declared war on Germany.

"The true aim of medicine is not to make men virtuous; it is to safeguard and rescue them from the consequences of their vices."
-Henry Louis Mencken

The series of articles that propelled Baltimore iconoclast H.L. Mencken to national fame, covering the Scopes "Monkey Trial," was still eleven years in the future when the journalist joined other writers and editors at a meeting of the Baltimore City Medical Society on April 7, 1914 to craft an agreement by which newspapers would develop their policy regarding medical reporting. Any publication of a physician's name in the papers, especially if it reported on a medical procedure, was deemed by the Society to be unprofessional.

Perhaps because he was, according to his friends, one of the worst hypochondriacs of his day, Mencken's presence at the meeting was not as risky as it may have been at a religious revival, a seance, or perhaps a political rally. He readily admitted his hypochondria, writing in 1926 "I have yet to meet an author who was not a hypochondriac. Saving only medical men, who are always ill and in fear of death, the literati are perhaps the most lavish consumers of pills and philtres in this world, and the most assiduous customers of surgeons. I cannot think of one, known to me personally, who is not constantly dosing himself with medicines, or regularly resorting to the knife."

Mencken, who liked nothing greater than to reveal a "buncomb...quack....a fraud...poppycock," found little to skewer in applied medicine, but much to pillory in its less-than-traditional offshoots. Of chiropractors he once wrote, after chortling over their contention that all of life's ills emanate from a pinched nerve, "The chiropractic therapeutics rest upon the doctrine that the way to get rid of such pinches is to climb upon a table and submit to a heroic pummeling by a retired piano mover." Chiropractors inadvertently served one purpose, however. They nearly put osteopaths out of business. In the face of the competition, Mencken reported in 1924 that osteopathy schools "now harry their students furiously, and turn them out ready for anything from growing hair on a bald head to frying a patient with the x-rays."

HLM regarded science in a different light, because it was based upon verifiable fact rather than faith, puffery and "hocus-pocus." Partly due to the influence of his mentor, Aldous Huxley, he zealously defended Darwinian evolution, perhaps no more floridly than in his dispatches to the *American Mercury* in 1925,while covering the infamous Scopes trial: "The Yahoos of the state of Tennessee have a clear right to have their progeny taught whatever they chose, and kept secure from whatever knowledge violated their superstitions."

Medicine also provided, for Mencken, another opportunity to point out the extraordinary level of ignorance of the American public (and at the same time extend collateral praise to the physician). "In the case of the American multitude," he wrote, the "accumulation of errors is of astounding bulk and consequence." In *The American Credo*, he accused the man in the street (*without* his tongue in his cheek) of believing that 1) "A doctor's family never gets sick," 2) "Surgeons often kill patients for the sheer fun of it," 3) "A doctor knows so much about women that he can no longer fall in love with one of them," 4) "All doctors intentionally write their prescriptions illegibly," 5) "Appendicitis is an ailment invented by surgeons years ago for moneymaking purposes," and 6) "When a doctor finds there is nothing the matter with a man who has come to consult with him, he never frankly tells the man that nothing is wrong, but gives him bread pills." Buncomb.

Baltimore City Medical Society Members go to War

Throughout 1917 and 1918 the medical challenges of modern warfare dominated the agenda of the Baltimore City Medical Society. Members were eager to learn of medical advances on the field of battle, and entertained presentations on a wide variety of technical topics. Many had direct application in civilian life, including "Modern Methods of Army Sanitation," and "Environmental Control of Military Camps and Stations."

As more Baltimore physicians enlisted and moved from their

surgeries to the Front, the question of providing for their patients in their absence was addressed. At the March 30, 1917 meeting, it was "Resolved that the Baltimore City Medical Society recognizes the patriotism of those members of the medical profession resident in Maryland who volunteer for service of the U.S. Government...in appreciation of this it is recommended that should these members of the profession be called to active service, the physicians who shall attend their patients should turn over one-third of the fees they collect from such patients to the physicians in active service or their families." The resolution was approved unanimously.

Even before Armistice, Society members had opportunities to hear first hand accounts from the front. Colonel C. K. Morgan, of the British Army Medical Service, spoke on "Medical and other Experiences on the Western Battle Front," and Sir Arthur Pearson presented "Work at St. Dunstan's Hospital for Blinded Soldiers." Speakers talked about surgical work in evacuation hospitals, the treatment and prevention of venereal disease among soldiers, the incidence and treatment of skin disease in the trenches, as well as general patriotic topics.

Almost as if the war experiences had opened the Society's eyes to a wider world, and as post-war meetings naturally shifted in focus from military to civilian topics, a number of international presentations began to appear in the Minutes in 1919. Members formally related their experiences not only in France during wartime, but in other foreign medical settings. Dr. J. Preston Maxwell accompanied his talk on "Medical Experiences of Twenty Years in China" with stereopticon slides. In December, 1920, Dr. Harry Friedenwald reflected upon his travels in the Middle East and spoke in particular about sanitary conditions in Palestine.

These lessons from the battlefield as well as the experiences gained from international travel and speakers from abroad had immediate application in the area of public health. Though Society meetings still featured nuts-and-bolts talks about the challenges faced by a physician in private practice on a daily basis, more time and resources were spent on topics of municipal sanitation, water treatment and waste removal, the quality of the local milk supply, and the provision for health care for the working and lower classes of Baltimore residents. Gradually, the Baltimore City Medical Society became less a venue to discuss particular medical problems and treatments and more an advocacy organization to do what the Preamble to the 1904 Constitution and By-Laws laid out as one of its missions: "elevate professional standards and improve public health conditions." The earlier efforts to properly label patent medicines served both purposes, and as early as 1908 the Society talked about whether unsanitary water was a vector for typhoid fever. In December, 1910, the Society held a symposium to ask the questions "What is Baltimore Doing for her Acutely Insane...her sufferers from acute infectious diseases...her tuberculosis patients...her alcoholics...her water supply?" The public health mission was established before World War I, and the Society returned to it as soon as the Armistice was signed.

Addressing Doctor-Nurse Responsibilities and Relations

Also in 1910, the Society began to examine the relationships between physicians, patients and nurses, though no conclusions were reached until 1917. Miss Mary E. Lent, who was the superintendent of the Visiting Nurses Association, read a paper entitled "District Nursing and What it Means to the Community" at the February 18, 1910 meeting. Sharing the agenda with Miss Lent that evening was Miss Eliza McLean, who asked the members to assist her in compiling a central directory of Baltimore nurses, to be maintained in the Faculty Building. An effort was to be made to combine the directories of twelve independent nursing associations across the city into a single source. The director of the Tuberculosis Nurses for the Baltimore City Health Department presented a talk on "The Neglected Tuberculosis Child."

But it was another seven years before the Society again turned its attention to the role of nurses, by establishing a committee to meet with the head of the Visiting Nurses Association "to bring into fuller harmony, relations between the members of the medical profession in Baltimore and the nurses of the Nurses Association." The committee concluded that while "harmonious" described most of their interactions, there had been "misunderstandings" because there was no clear, published description of the functions of nurses. That the errors were caused by the nursing community was made abundantly clear by the Society, as was the opinion that "members of the medical profession" did not include nurses.

The concern was that the nurses sometimes "encroached upon the province of the attending physician," when in fact their responsibility was limited to carrying out the doctor's instructions to the letter. A regimen of Standing Orders for Nurses was devised, which while described as "a few simple rules" in fact was a detailed list of what the nurse should do in various cases not only to better serve the patient but to reinforce the role of the attending physician.

"Where the family can afford to hire a private physician, the nurse shall try to see to it that only one physician is in charge...When the family cannot afford a physician, the nurse may call in any of the physicians attached to the nearest City Hospital agency or Dispensary." In the absence of a doctor from one of the city facilities the nurse, after "having made every reasonable effort" may call upon a private practitioner, but "only such private physicians...as have indicated a willingness to cooperate with the district nurse by calling on patients for her free of charge."

Among the Standing Orders by which the nurse was regulated, most limited her to functions like preparing baths and ordering the sick room "with special emphasis on good ventilation, cleanliness..." She was permitted to mop with disinfectant, apply dressings, cleanse wounds, boil drinking water, administer enemas and mouthwashes. An important part of the job was advising patients about cleanliness and diet. She did not administer medications or inoculations, and was admonished to take no initiative beyond "prop[ping] up with a pillow" and calling the primary physician.

In the modern era, when the rationing of health care is reality in many places, when the escalating cost of care is one of the industry's greatest challenges, and in which nurses are called upon for an ever-widening array of procedures, it is strange to recall that just two generations past the nurse's duty was limited to handing the syringe to the doctor and doing alcohol rubs.

Post-War Politics and Medicine

By 1920, the Baltimore City Medical Society had grown to 720 members. The first resolution of the new decade was in honor of Dr. Sir William Osler, who died at Oxford, England on December 29, 1919:

> "Physician, teacher, guide, lover of his fellow man. Noble exemplar of charity and tolerance and temperance and work and love. Untiring stimulator and generous benefactor of this Society, whose sparkling wit and genial, subtle humor smoothed the rough way of life for so many weary spirits; Whose presence banished discord and suspicion. The gap which his absence leaves among us will forever be warmed by the glow of that all-embracing love which radiated from his presence like a halo of light."

The end of World War I allowed the Society to turn its attention to a wide range of local health initiatives. The group regularly voted to support bond issues for new hospitals and clean drinking water. It spoke out against political maneuvering in issues of medical importance, rejecting, for example, an effort to move the Board of Medical Examiners to the Department of Employment and

Registration, fearing that such a move would politicize the Board. In the mayoral election of 1923, the Society urged that every candidate follow the example of Howard Jackson in declaring that the "Health Department, in the event of this candidate's election, shall be kept clear of politics, and that the Health Commissioner to be appointed shall be the most competent municipal health administrator procurable, regardless of party affiliation."

Howard Jackson won that election, and it was to his office in City Hall that the Society directed a letter in April, 1927, that reported on the work of its Joint Committee on Municipal Ambulances. The subject of a public ambulance service had arisen the year before, when a paper entitled "The Need for an Emergency Ambulance Service in Baltimore" was presented and the committee established. There were sporadic reports on the committee's progress, and the 1927 letter followed six talks about ambulances and emergency service. A Resolution was read into the proceedings:

> "RESOLVED: That the plan submitted by the Joint Committee on Municipal Ambulances to Mayor Howard W. Jackson, is heartily indorsed by the joint meeting of the component societies. The care of the sick and injured is strictly a medical matter, therefore, the responsibility rests upon the HOSPITALS and the City of Baltimore for ambulance service, and upon no other agency."

Drawn by a committee composed of members of the Baltimore City Medical Society, the West Baltimore Medical Society, the Baltimore Association of Commerce and the Baltimore Safety Council, the plan was detailed. It called for the appropriation of $21,000 for the purchase of seven ambulances and $45,000 for the annual operation of the emergency service. Initially, the presence of a nurse on each ambulance was suggested, but that was dropped. The most contentious part of the proposal was that the service be run by the Supervisor of City Charities (the modern welfare department) and that the ambulances be stationed at and operated by hospitals, and manned by trained hospital personnel.

Of the eleven hospitals that responded to the request for support from the Society, five came with the full "indorsement of the Committee's aim and entire sympathy with the plan." Their support, however, came with the caveat that although they thought the service a good idea, they could not operate an ambulance or accept patients "owing to a lack of ward beds, especialized nature of the work or non-admission of colored patients." Six others agreed only to accept patients delivered to them by the ambulance service, stopping short of complete endorsement.

Regardless of the structure of the service, it was a pioneering effort. Prior to the first Baltimore City ambulance's rolling onto the streets, patients were transported in police patrol wagons. Other cities either failed to address the problem at all or did so decades after it was settled in Baltimore. Typically, the local funeral director provided transportation services, which could have in no way been a psychological encouragement to the patient thus being taken to the hospital. But hearses were designed to transport a horizontal body and mortuary staffs were accustomed to handling bodies. South Carolina continued to tolerate patients carried in hearses until 1974, stopping only at the insistence of the 1973 Emergency Medical Services Act. Police still carried patients to hospitals in what they insensitively called a "scoop and haul" system. The city of New Bedford established the first public ambulance service in Massachusetts in 1976, almost half a century after Baltimore.

"I shall make arrangements at once for the operation of five ambulances under the supervision of the Fire Department."
-Mayor Howard W. Jackson
April 23, 1927

With the establishment of the first public ambulance service in Baltimore, the city fathers (at the urging of the Baltimore City Medical Society) demonstrated that they had learned the lesson that prompt response to medical crises saves lives. There were private services on city streets by then, but the only example anywhere of anything even remotely resembling a universal service came during wartime. Battlefield ambulances were nothing new, and their efficiency served as a model for civilian operations.

At least it can be said that among the dreadful aftermaths of war are usually found accelerated advances in medical practice. Until the late 15th Century, when King Ferdinand and Queen Isabella of Spain accompanied their troops on crusades against the Moors, if a soldier were wounded in battle he was pretty much left to his own devices. There were crude horse litters to remove the wounded from the field of battle, but they seldom arrived on the scene until hours, or perhaps days, after the last arrow was fired.

Ferdinand and Isabella established the first military hospitals, called *ambulancias*. Three centuries later, Dominique-Jean Larrey devised the first real battlefield ambulance service as he accompanied Napoleon's troops across Prussia. His two-wheeled wagons - "flying ambulances" - allowed the surgeon to work on the battlefield and dramatically lowered mortality.

Larrey's ambulances were adapted for civilian use, and the notion of treating the ill or wounded while they were on their way to the hospital caught on. In 1832, a carriage for cholera patients was invented that warmed the patient on a mattress of heated salt. "The curative process commences the instant the patient is put into the carriage; time is saved which can be given to the care of the patient..." the *London Medical Gazette* commented.

At the outbreak of the American Civil War, surgeon Jonathan Letterman was assigned to the Army of the Potomac, and by 1862 he determined that the flimsy "Two-Wheeled Finley" ambulance was not up to the task. Letterman not only invented an improved wagon, he also reorganized the ambulance service that provided for an effective field hospital and an expeditious system of transport of the wounded. During the war, the Geneva Convention of 1864 was drafted (in response to battlefield conditions observed by Florence Nightingale in the Crimean War of 1854-1856). The Convention provided for the neutrality of ambulances and established the universal symbol of the red cross on a white background that still identifies emergency vehicles.

These developments led to the establishment of private civilian ambulance services in major cities. The Commercial Hospital (now Cleveland General) boasts the first ambulance service in America, which began transporting patients in 1865. Bellevue Hospital's carriages serviced the entire city of New York by 1869. With the establishment of the American Red Cross in 1884, Clara Barton's wartime experiences with the United States Sanitary Commission were translated into preparation for disaster relief for civilians, including plans for effective transportation.

War has continued to be an important impetus for the improvement of patient transport. Motorized ambulances received their first test under fire during World War I, and as a result most civilian ambulance services that still relied on horses moved to the automobile after the troops returned. After the "War to End All Wars", airplane ambulances were developed, leading eventually to the helicopter ambulances of Korea and Vietnam and the adaptation of the same aircraft to civilian shock-trauma scenarios.

Baltimore's Mayor Jackson politely received the 1927 proposal of the Committee and promised it his careful consideration. He concluded, however, that the service would be best put under the control of the Fire Department, not the City Charities Department. His statement of April 23, 1927, pointed to the experience of firefighters in responding to emergencies, and divided the city into five districts. The Fire Department was ordered to determine which station houses were best located in each district, and to train at least 20 firefighters in first aid. The service was to be under the control of a surgeon who would be responsible for the training, record keeping, and when required, his medical expertise.

"It is conceded that the great need is for a service that will get the patient to the hospital as quickly as possible. The well-recognized promptness of the Fire Department, their training to answer emergency calls and their ability to get to the scene of the trouble with all possible speed, make it certain that they will be able to render service that could not possibly be obtained through other agencies," Mayor Jackson said in an April, 1927 press release.

The Mayor's plan took the control of the service out of the hands of the hospitals and physicians. The latter were split on the wisdom of the Fire Department's involvement. Dr. A.G. Barrett, President of the West Baltimore Medical Society, said in the April 24, 1927 *Sun*, "He should have placed the ambulance service under the hospitals where they could have functioned efficiently from the start."

Dr. Winford H. Smith, Chief of Surgery at Johns Hopkins Hospital, supported the continuation of emergency services under the auspices of the Police Department, using modern emergency vehicles. He reported that an investigation of cities that subsidized public ambulance services and left the operation to individual hospitals showed that the hospitals eventually abandoned the plan because "it became a nuisance."

"Another weakness of the plan," he continued, "is that Baltimore has no great City Hospital always ready to take in patients. Many of the institutions here do not take colored patients at all, others take only male ones. If the plan were to work at all...there would have to be some understanding between hospitals." Baltimore's population was almost a third African-American in the 1920 census.

Baltimore City wasted no time in deploying its ambulances, purchasing three Studebakers and two Buicks in June, 1927 and assigning one to each of five districts. These ambulances were to be called from the same street boxes used to summon the fire department. Patients were to be removed "only...from the public highways," and "not in the cases of violence; police patrol wagons must be used for that purpose." In the first year, those five ambulances responded to 8,222 calls.

Ambulances did not dominate the Society's agenda as the nation was swept through the Roaring Twenties. The group addressed many other issues. Also in 1927, a resolution stated "that a Psychopathic Hospital for the City of Baltimore is an absolute necessity," and urged the City of Baltimore to establish one. At the same meeting, one of two important Bills before both the Maryland State Senate and House of Delegates was discussed, a move by the state's Christian Scientists to exempt them from the provisions of the Medical Practice Act. The Society was especially incensed by the possibility that "faith healing" may be recognized as medicine. The effort failed, but was reborn two years later, and in February, 1929, the Society received a letter from the Chairman of the Maryland Medical and Chirurgical Faculty Legislative Committee, Dr. Josiah S. Bowen: "While this Bill is designed to permit 'Christian Science practitioners or healers to charge and collect fees for their ministration by spiritual or mental means', it is so worded that it would open the gates to any charlatan or pow-wow who would claim to be 'practicing the religious tenets of his church'."

An issue of more immediate medical importance, a threat to the "dignity of the profession," was the potential elevation of osteopaths to full medical recognition. Osteopathy, considered a close cousin of chiropractic care, was condemned along with homeopathy and snake oil. A Maryland House of Delegates Bill introduced in the 1927 session would have granted to osteopaths the privilege of conducting all surgery except "major" surgery (which was not defined in the Bill's language). It conferred on the osteopath the right to prescribe drugs. A letter to the Society from Dr. F.V. Beitler, Chief of the city's Bureau of Vital Statistics, called the Bill "the poorest drawn Bill and the vaguest piece of English that I have seen in a long time." Because osteopaths failed nearly every criteria used to qualify as physicians, few had formal medical or surgical training beyond the most cursory, and because the Bill did not require them to pass the same examination as doctors, the Society objected. The Bill died.

That same year the Society considered assuming the role of coordinator of a program of post-graduate courses to be created by hospitals whose specialties made a topic a particularly good fit. A committee had been appointed to study the practical facilities for Graduate Medical Teaching in Baltimore. The committee's report claimed that "There can be little question, however, that the hospitals of Baltimore would be greatly strengthened if each one attempted to develop some feature of its work to the point where it would be useful for the teaching of post-graduates." The report was read into the Minutes, and a vote cast on a proposal to create a committee to catalog graduate programs at various hospitals. The motion failed to receive a second, and the meeting proceeded to the evening's scientific topics.

Thus the Society moved beyond the crash of the stock market on Black Friday, in October, 1929 and into the years of the Depression. The same agenda prevailed at most meetings, standing committee reports followed by special issues, usually legislative, with the meeting closing after a series of scientific talks (often as many as 4 in a single semi-monthly meeting). There were 744 members as the nation's economy began its long decline, and a deficit in the bank account of $270.19 (a healthier balance just two years earlier stood at $1,705.55). In 1930 the dues were increased to $20 annually to restore the bank account to the black. A former President of the Baltimore City Medical Society, Dr. William S. Thayer, had risen to the Presidency of the American Medical Association.

There is almost no mention in the Society's records of the effect of rising unemployment, bank failures and bread lines on the City throughout the years leading to World War II. Baltimore City instituted a campaign to innoculate against diphtheria and the Society signed on wholeheartedly in 1932. In 1934, the Society in partnership with several other local groups formed the Baltimore Hospital Service Association to offer pre-paid hospitalization insurance through employers to lower and middle income Baltimoreans. The Association got off to a rocky start (see more in the chapter on health care economics), but the influence of the Society kept it going. A Pediatric Section was established, and the Society participated in a study of maternal mortality in Baltimore.

Membership rebounded to 863 by 1935, and the bank balance had regained its healthy position, showing $620.13 as the year opened. For the first time in its history, the Society embarked on an examination of the practice of calling "expert" medical witnesses to testify in court, and the state Faculty's Legal Committee, working with the Baltimore Bar Association, drew up legislation to control the mechanism by which witnesses were chosen. The problems surrounding testimony were considered. That witnesses' statements were so often controversial and so technical as to be useless to a judge and a jury of the defendant's peers was pointed out. In some cases, the physician on the stand was so prejudiced on behalf of one party or the other that "he becomes an advocate instead of a witness." Finally, it was observed that sometimes the witness was so biased in the favor of the plaintiff that the desire for the correct verdict overcame the necessity of truthfulness.

The collaboration of the legal and medical communities resulted in a Bill giving courts the power to assign expert witnesses to cases who were not connected to either plaintiff or defendant. It established a method by which flagrant violations of the standards would be referred to the Medical and Chirurgical Faculty for examination. In order to prepare students to deal with ethical matters, the Bill called for each major medical school to begin courses in medical ethics, and that hospitals be encouraged to offer continuing education courses in ethics to their staffs. In February, 1938, the Honorable Eugene O'Dunne of the Supreme Bench of Baltimore City delivered an address at a Society meeting entitled "The Medical Man on the Witness Stand."

In October, 1940, as the nation watched Europe in chaos, the Society voted to allow members of the Monumental City Medical Society, the city's professional organization for African American physicians, to attend any technical or scientific presentation at a Baltimore City Medical Society meeting. As the new decade

THE BALTIMORE CITY MEDICAL SOCIETY - A History

opened, the international crisis began to intercede on the Society's orderly agendas. Ten months before America's entry into World War II the Society welcomed Dr. Joseph Stokes of the University of Pennsylvania to talk about his recent experiences as a physician in France. The director of the Selective Service System in Maryland addressed an October, 1941 meeting about the medical defects commonly found in draftees, and the public health implications of those problems. At the following meeting there were no civilian scientific topics. Instead, Dr. John Davis talked about the treatment of wounds, and the Baltimore City Health Commissioner spoke of his experiences in London in wartime.

Two days before the attack on Pearl Harbor, the Baltimore City Medical Society met for its 37th Annual Meeting. Membership was steady at 847, and the bank balance stood at $4252.07. Most meetings for the next four years were dominated by talk of the medical exigencies of modern warfare - medicine in civilian defense, treatment of chemical warfare casualties, gasoline and tire rationing as it affected medical service, war neuroses and clinical aspects of tropical diseases. The increase in membership throughout the war years - 908 at the end of 1942, 938 a year later, and 970 as the last year of the war opened - made note of the fact that many were on active duty. Over a quarter of the Society's members were serving in military capacities in 1944. During World War II, 718 doctors served in the armed forces from Maryland - 577 of those practiced in Baltimore City before the war.

"At the conclusion of the meeting, the President called attention to the fact that a new ship was to be christened **Sir William Osler** *on the following day, in Baltimore. He felt that such an announcement was especially appropriate in Osler Hall on the occasion of a program having to do with marine medical problems."*

-Samuel M. McLanahan, M.D.
writing in the March 5, 1943 Minutes of
the Baltimore City Medical Society.
The President to whose comments
he quoted was Walter D. Wise, M.D.

"Problems in the care of shipwrecked personnel in lifeboats," by Surgeon Commander E.W. Musson, M.D."

-the program to which Dr. McLanahan referred above
March 5, 1943

"The policy of the American Medical Association is to admit members regardless of race, color or creed. The majority of constituent state medical associations admit colored physicians to membership...The exception to this is the constituent associations in the states in the South. Where these physicians are not admitted some of the southern states' medical associations are very anxious to work out some scheme whereby these men may become members."

-from a December 7, 1948 letter from the AMA to Dr. Alexander J. Schaffer, Baltimore City Medical Society

"A Stand for Democracy Within the Medical Profession"

-Dr. W. Horsley Gantt, Chairman
Baltimore City Medical Society Committee on Admission of
Negro Physicians
October, 1948

The Baltimore City Medical Society Enters the Post-World War II Years

As Allied forces closed in on Berlin in the spring of 1945, war still raged in the Pacific and the need for physicians was unabated. So on March 16th of that year, with the end of the war in sight, the Office of Naval Officer Procurement in Washington wrote to the Baltimore City Medical Society, expressing its anxiety at being able to field so few physicians. This was the last entry in the Society's Minutes that referred to World War II before the atomic bomb put an abrupt end to fighting.

Returning doctors immediately took an active role in the Society's proceedings, and like those before them who came back to civilian life from the battlefield, they brought the lessons of warfare with them. There was something different this time, however. There was the sense that if America could defeat the combined Axis powers there was no challenge that was beyond the nation's ability to meet. A sense of optimism pervaded; soldiers and sailors were greeted upon their return with the GI Bill to provide education and to fund home ownership. Talk of providing medical care to everyone arose again in Washington. What would become the Civil Rights Movement of the fifties and sixties began to form its credo. The Marshall Plan, largely an American initiative, rebuilt the societies and economies of former enemies, a radical humanitarian departure from the close of the previous war, when only retribution and discipline were sought.

"We know that under it [liberty] we can meet the hard problems of peace which have come upon us. A free people with free Allies, who can develop an atomic bomb, can use the same skill and energy and determination to overcome all the difficulties ahead...But we face the future and all its dangers with great confidence and great hope. America can build for itself a future of employment and security," President Harry Truman said from the White House on the occasion of the Japanese surrender.

There was an urgency to get back to the business of running the country, an urgency reflected in the post-war Minutes of the

Baltimore City Medical Society. Twenty-five years earlier, when their fathers returned from World War I, the agenda of the Society was more crowded with reminiscences of trench medicine, and wartime experiences were related at general meetings for nearly three years. This time, the younger generation was anxious to put the war behind them and to turn their attention to what they correctly anticipated was going to be a challenging and exciting period in the history of medicine in Baltimore.

"Write lots about it. Go clear overboard for it, say that plasma is the outstanding medical discovery of this war."
-US Army surgeons, talking to reporter Ernie Pyle
Sicily, 1943

World War II was the first major battlefield trial of plasma, first made by American physicians in 1930 from the separation of red and white blood cells. Plasma proved to be a sound replacement for whole blood, which deteriorated after only a few days in storage. The availability of plasma made blood transfusions practical for severe injuries outside the normal hospital setting, and expanded the understanding of blood transfusion as a tool to combat wound shock, an important discovery of the previous World War. Dr. Charles Drew, who had already revolutionized blood distribution by creating a blood bank at New York's Columbia Medical Center in 1938, was called upon to organize the first American Red Cross Blood Bank. Under his leadership, an efficient means of collecting and preserving plasma was developed and became a model for civilian blood banks after the war.

When US Army Surgeon John Currey sent a cavalryman or an Army of the Potomac infantryman to the rear following battlefield surgery in the Civil War, that trooper's chance of survival was only 50%. During World War II, 85% of the soldiers who underwent front line surgery survived. Fewer than 4% of all wounded soldiers who were treated at field hospitals died. This remarkable recovery rate was largely the result of improved medical transport and well-organized treatment, based in part on modern assembly line techniques learned from American industry. The medics were a wounded soldier's first contact with medical care, and they were equipped with morphine, plasma and sulfanilamide. Most were transported quickly to a battalion aid station, where they were stabilized for the next leg of the trip, to a collecting station. Surgery was performed at collecting stations and wounded were prepared for the short trip to a clearing station or field hospital, usually within 40 miles of the front. Reporter Ernie Pyle wrote home about a field hospital where he spent just one day - and moved three times. The further from the front, the larger and more sophisticated the hospitals became until the gravest patients found themselves on board massive hospital ships off the coast of Africa.

This war, like all that came before it, proved to be the ultimate testing ground for recent developments, in this case "wonder drugs" like penicillin and sulfanilamide as well as plasma. In the months prior to the attack on Pearl Harbor, the amazing ability of penicillin to attack a wide variety of bacteria was recognized, but there was no mechanism to produce it in the volume that global war would require. American pharmaceutical giant Pfizer began experimentation with mass production techniques in 1942, eventually allowing 19 other firms to make penicillin using its process. At the outbreak of hostilities it was only possible to manufacture penicillin in lots of a few hundred doses at a time, but by D-Day improved methods made it possible to have an adequate supply available to field hospitals to treat every casualty. One of the most important legacies of the war, penicillin was widely available to the post-war civilian public and its discoverer, bacteriologist Sir Andrew Fleming, received the 1945 Nobel prize.

Wartime conditions hastened the advancement of treatment for burns. Because of the reliance on tanks, as well as the development of large armored personnel carriers, the incidence of burn wounds skyrocketed. A burning personnel carrier became an oven when hit, and abandoning it was slow and difficult. Medics treated burns with gauze pads impregnated with jelly and sulfa drugs, which was much more effective than the tannic acid methods used in World War I. As a result, pain and infection were greatly reduced.

Countless other developments were either used for the first time in World War II, or used for the first time on a large scale. The drug Atarban proved effective in treating malaria in the Pacific theatre (World War II was the first war in which disease did not take more lives than violence). DDT, since abandoned because of the environmental consequences of its use, saved many human lives by killing animal disease vectors. The invention of morphine "syrettes", single-dose injectors, revolutionized drug delivery systems and laid the groundwork for similar applications in civilian hospitals.

Among the earliest efforts to return to normality was the dismissal of two Society committees that served throughout the duration of the war. During the Annual Meeting, four years to the day after the attack on Pearl Harbor, the Society closed the books on the War Price and Rationing Board Committee and the Civilian Mobilization Committee. Dr. J.M.H. Rowland, chair of the former and Dr. Frederick B. Smith who presided over the latter were thanked for their work. Two hundred and twenty-eight of the 1028 members were still on active duty. One year later, at the end of 1946, only 91 active members had yet to return to civilian life.

When Dr. Alexander Schaffer returned from the Far East he described his experiences battling malaria, and at the same regular meeting in early January, 1946, Dr. Lewis P. Gundry, who in 8 years would be elected to the Society's presidency, talked about his own service in the Pacific. Among the veterans were the future leaders of the Society. Dr. Harry M. Robinson, Jr., who became the 65th president in 1969, concluded this same 1946 meeting with an illustrated presentation on "Some Dermatological Problems in the Tropics." Succeeding topics included "Medical Problems in the North African and Mediterranean Theatres of Operations," "The

Developing Program for the Care of the Veteran," "Five Hundred and Twenty-Three Acute War Wounds of the Abdomen," and "Combat Injuries of the Colon." Except for a single slide presentation about medical care in occupied Germany in 1949, the last war-related talk was delivered in October, 1946, scarcely a year after arms were laid down. The Baltimore City Medical Society was poised to put the war to rest and move forward.

"The achievements and sacrifices of our African American Physicians are so often overlooked. They have faced and crossed the barriers [from which] many would have turned away."
-Trudy R. Hall, M.D., President
Monumental City Medical Society
from a letter to members, November, 2003

The Monumental City Medical Society and its Forebears

The *First Colored Professional, Clerical and Business Directory of Baltimore City*, in its 1913 first edition, listed the officers of the Baltimore Medical Association. This is the first published mention of a medical society for African American practitioners in Baltimore. Its President was Howard E. Young, M.D. By the next year, a companion society formed, the Maryland Medical Dental and Pharmaceutical Association, with Dr. Young, who continued as President of the Baltimore association, at its helm. It was not until 1949 that African American physicians were granted full membership in the Baltimore City Medical Society.

Records of the early African American professional groups are sketchy, but both the state and local organization were listed separately in the directory until 1923, when the Baltimore Medical Association disappeared. By 1929 the group had grown substantially enough that a president was required for each of the three disciplines. Dr. Young served as President of the Pharmaceutical Association, Dr. J.G. McRae presided over the Medical Association, and Dr. Oliver W.H. McNeil was the President of the Dental Association. Dr. Young remained in his position until the creation of the Monumental City Medical Society.

A group of physicians, dentists and pharmacists convened in 1928 to form the Me-De-So Club. Initially a reading group, it evolved into a medical professional society that explored issues critical to the black community in not only medical, but also social and cultural arenas. Me-De-So, as it celebrated its 56th year in 2004, continued to be a vital part of the community, having built an 88-unit apartment complex and having its work supplemented by an active auxiliary. Its members have always been active in the Monumental City Medical Society.

Since its inception, Monumental City Medical Society has been a local component of the National Medical Association. Founded in 1895, the NMA is the nation's oldest professional society representing African American physicians and health care providers. It was created after African American applicants had repeatedly been rejected by the AMA, at a time when racial disparity relegated most black Americans to sub-standard hospitals manned by overworked staff.

Only two segregated schools conferred M.D. degrees, Howard University in Washington, D.C. and the Meharry Medical College in Nashville.

The Monumental City Medical Society pursued the same goals as its white counterpart society: licensure of physicians and maintenance of professional standards, continuing education, legislation and public health efforts. Because its members faced daunting barriers of medical school admission, hospital access, government indifference and economic hardship, its mission was and continues to be more targeted to the health care issues of minorities. It was not until 1885 that the first hospital in Baltimore that freely admitted black citizens was opened, Dr. G.W. Kennard's Hospital on Ensor Street. Provident Hospital, the first African American owned hospital in America, opened in Baltimore in 1894. The University of Maryland School of Medicine admitted its first African American student in 1951, with Hopkins not following suit until 1963.

During Dr. Allan D. Jensen's BCMS Presidency in 1992, the partnership between the societies was strengthened. Dr. Willarda V. Edwards served concurrently as president of both organizations in 1995. The result of the flourishing relationship was an ongoing series of joint meetings and programs that are well-attended.

Among the Society's centerpiece programs is its scholarship program. Begun in 1990, the scholarship conferred $108,500 in aid to deserving medical students in its first 13 years. The Society's programs in Continuing Medical Education and its practice enhancement seminars address the particular needs of African American practitioners.

Two years later, in 1948, the Society addressed what would become the most crucial issue in domestic American history of the final half of the twentieth century. The admission of African American physicians had already been tabled by the state Faculty, and sent to the constituent local assemblies for a decision. Because Baltimore was a magnet for black Americans leaving the fields of the South for the factories of the North, and because the state's African American population was largely settled in the city, perhaps the issue of integration of the City Society was more urgent than for the more distant counties. Members of the Monumental City Medical Society, Baltimore's equivalent of the Baltimore City Medical Society for black physicians, had been officially welcome at technical and scientific meetings since 1940. In any case, the Society determined to move forward boldly.

Dr. W. Horsley Gantt, who crafted the Society's policy regarding integration of its membership, was clear in his opinion: "The Committee feels that in a professional body, organized for the advancement of clinical and scientific medicine, that its educational function should be made accessible to as many physicians as possible, and that there should be no prohibition to membership of any physicians who are eligible professionally."

Baltimore was still, in 1948, very much a segregated city. Jim Crow laws still dictated who could ride where on public transportation, sit at what lunch counter and shop in which department stores. African Americans had to picket Ford's Theatre for seven years before finally being admitted in 1952. Marian Anderson, who performed at the Lyric Theatre in 1953, could not find a hotel room in Baltimore. In 1955, when the Society was pushing to host the Southern Medical Association's 1958 Annual Meeting, their colleagues in the South expressed reservations about the social functions. It was determined that while all members of the Baltimore City Medical Society would be invited to scientific sessions, invitations to social affairs would be sent individually, which would "obviate any embarrassment to our colored members." On this basis the Society decided that it was acceptable to invite the southern members to Baltimore. The Southern Medical Association, though probably unconcerned about the feelings of black physicians in Baltimore, decided to go elsewhere.

Not every member was enthusiastically supportive of Dr. Gantt's position. Some admitted reluctantly that it was an issue that had to be faced. One physician felt "that we should wait until the City program for the care of the indigent sick has had a further trial; the hope being that this work, carried out by both white and colored physicians, may give a clue as to how such racial cooperation will work out." Others expressed concern about the social gatherings. Ultimately, in 1949 the Society voted unanimously in favor of unlimited admission to African American physicians, becoming the first society south of the Mason Dixon Line to do so.

The Society's decision brought it national acclaim in 1950, when the Sidney Hollander Foundation honored the Baltimore City Medical Society for "an outstanding contribution toward the achievement of equal rights and opportunities for Negroes in Maryland." The presentation was made by Dr. Arthur O. Lovejoy, Professor Emeritus of Philosophy at Johns Hopkins University. Dr. Lovejoy's words conveyed the progressive importance of the event:

> "...these awards...are made in recognition of actions contributory to what is called 'the improvement in human relations.' For, next to the saving of life itself, and the raising of the level of physical and mental health in individuals - which is *your* great special function in the economy of the modern society - the chief business of mankind is the improvement of human relations...In the present stage of terrestrial history, human relations are, one is tempted to think, in a more deplorable and tragic state than they ever have been before...in this strange, dark scene

there appear, here and there, new lights - little lights perhaps in themselves, but evidences that men are also seeking and learning to live in more kindly, more cooperative, more brotherly relations with other men...such a light was lit in Baltimore when the City Medical Society resolved to admit Negro physicians to participation in the privileges of membership."

The only unfortunate part of the landmark evening, April 21, 1950, was that the microphone at the podium failed. So the Society had 600 copies of Dr. Lovejoy's speech printed and mailed to members.

Emergency Medical Services and the Society's Response

At the same time that the Society was opening its doors to African American colleagues, it was working to extend access to medical care, especially in the case of emergency, by creating an emergency telephone response service. Anyone who was in dire need of a doctor's care, but unable to reach a doctor, could talk to a trained operator by dialing Lexington 1000. The operator was prepared with a list of 200 physicians who had volunteered to be on call 24 hours a day. The list was organized by postal zones, and doctors moved up the list until they had fielded a call, after which their name was moved to the bottom of the list.

During a 17-day trial period in May, 1950, 91 calls were handled. In each case, the operator determined the whereabouts of the caller, whether it was indeed an emergency, and how payment would be made for the service. Then, putting the patient on hold, the operator called the doctor at the top of the list nearest to the patient's neighborhood. When the doctor was reached, the responsibility of the phone service ended. Should the patient be unable to pay privately for care, the operator was instructed to call the Fire Department (from which the municipal ambulance service was run) and between the ambulance service and the Welfare Doctor on call arrangements could quickly be made. In cases which were, in the opinion of the operator, of a life-and-death nature, an ambulance with a physician on board was immediately dispatched regardless of the prospect of a fee.

"LE 1000 is not just a number to obtain a doctor. It is to be used only in cases of genuine emergencies," Dr. Douglas Stone, who chaired the Society committee that prepared the service plan, advised readers of the *Sun* on May 25, 1950. The service included volunteer specialists as well as general practitioners, and was operated at no charge to the Society by the Physicians' Exchange, an answering service in the Court Square Building in downtown

Baltimore. The following month it was announced that the Baltimore Retail Druggists Association would offer round-the-clock access to a pharmacist. Six months after the first call was made, the "Medical Service", as it was called, had handled 199 cases, ranging from heart attacks to a child who swallowed a quarter.

By 1952 over 350 doctors and 140 pharmacists were volunteering. An average of ten calls daily came through the switchboard, and local hospitals reported that pressure on their emergency rooms had been relieved by the availability of the service. It can only be hoped that the ambulance attendants were successful in freeing the child whose frantic mother called the service to report that her son had become entangled in the wringer of her washing machine.

Call volume increased to nearly 4,000 in 1959, and the constant problem of enlisting volunteer physicians continued. With 130 volunteers on the list, that meant a doctor was likely to be called upon on average 31 times a year. As might be imagined, there was resentment among those volunteers who agreed to be awakened in the middle of the night for a case of appendicitis, while other practitioners who refused to participate stayed tucked warmly between the sheets. As early as 1953, a survey of emergency doctors revealed that "The complaint which occurs most often was the fact that men feel they should not be made to bear the brunt of handling night calls for men who are either unwilling to take their own emergency calls or who make no provisions for having their phones covered while they are not available."

A year earlier the Society had branded the reluctance of some doctors to go on emergency calls as "a practice...that is not only bad for the public relations of the medical profession, but exhibits a lack of the proper interest on the part of physicians concerning their patients." The Resolution went on to point out that medical ethics was taught in only a very "superficial and skimpy" fashion. A letter was drafted to the Deans of each of the two major medical schools to "see that more time and attention is paid...to teaching the ethics of our profession, the obligations of the Hippocratic oath." The short-term solution to the problem of providing willing physicians to handle emergency work was to encourage young physicians to add their names to the list, and these doctors seemed eager to gain the experience it offered.

For a second time, the Society in 1953 turned its attention to the necessity of providing formal postgraduate education for younger practitioners in Baltimore in addition to expanding their range of experiences by exposing them to the emergency needs of a major metropolitan center. The regular clinical and scientific sessions, of course, served a similar purpose, but there was a need for more organized curricula. Twenty-five years earlier, in 1928, a committee was established to study facilities for postgraduate medical education in Baltimore. It concluded that "The hospital situation in Baltimore at the present does not lend itself in any way to a general effort towards organized postgraduate teaching. With the exception of the two medical schools, ...no hospital attempts to have a routine attendance on the part of its clinical staff and in consequence no systematic teaching effort would be possible...Should it prove possible to organize a sufficient number of graduate courses in the various hospitals, the Baltimore City Medical Society might serve as a coordinating agency. An office might be maintained at which prospective students could receive information and be formally registered for the various courses. Such an office could also furnish to visiting physicians from the counties information in regard to the time and place of clinics and lectures in the various hospitals of the City."

Nothing came of the committee's report in 1927, but in December, 1953 the topic again arose and it was noted that the situation had not improved. That year a Committee on Postgraduate Education was re-instituted to fill the gap, and in its year end report it announced the creation of a course program that offered sessions on psychiatry, cardiology, pediatrics, dermatology and allergy. An ambitious program, the schedule called for courses to run the following January and February and again in the first 3 months of 1955. Dr. Harry M. Robinson, Jr., committee chairman, reported a year later that "The courses given in the first month have an average attendance of 108 men each night."

The Society in the 1950's

Amidst the routine matters that the Society addressed monthly (October through March only) throughout the decade of the 1950's, in addition to the scientific, educational and political agendas are found notations on other activities. Though the Minutes do not reveal the formation of a Women's Auxiliary in March, 1950, they do thank the Auxiliary annually for the various dinners and social functions it made possible, the educational initiatives it mounted and the ways in which it helped with other Society functions. At the end of that year the roll of members reached 1,376.

Beginning in 1952, meetings were frequently accompanied by "lantern slides," the result of a donation of two slide projectors by Charles P. McCormick, the Chief Executive Officer of McCormick Spice. Though the fight to prevent socialized medicine, defined by the Society as any form of government-mandated medical insurance, dominated the agendas in the following several years, the Society found time to lobby the State Legislature during the 1954 session to permit the sale of "non-fat milk preparations," which "are of value as a component of special diets which are recommended for the treatment of particular problems." It was illegal under laws controlling the sale of milk to sell anything but whole milk, but following the resolution of the Society, the Maryland State Health Department altered the regulations.

One of the big events in late 1953 was the announcement that the American League baseball team, the St. Louis Browns, was purchased by local interests and would be playing in Baltimore the following season as the Baltimore Orioles. The team asked the Baltimore City Medical Society in December of that year if it could have use of the Society's Addressograph machine, and access was granted provided that the Orioles pay their own expenses.

When the *Baltimore News Post* came to the Society requesting that a physician write a weekly question-and-answer column, along the lines of a similar service provided by the Philadelphia County Medical Society in the *Philadelphia Inquirer*, the matter was forwarded to Dr. Amos Koontz, Chairman of the Committee on Public Education. The columns began to appear in 1954, though not without some controversy. The decision to proceed was made by the Executive Committee, and when the membership was advised, Dr. Alan Chesney objected that this was "a move in the direction of medicine by correspondence." Dr. Koontz explained that the questions would be fielded by a Committee member, Dr. H. Hanford Hopkins, who would forward them to the members who could most capably answer them. That put the matter to rest.

That same year marked the beginning of a partnership with the Baltimore Council of Boy Scouts that lasted for many years. The Scouts asked if the Society would be willing to provide volunteer physicians to conduct physical examinations of the 400 boys who arrived at Broad Creek Scout Camp, in Harford County near Cardiff, Maryland, and to man the "Casualty Aid Stations" at several of the big summertime events. During the first summer, 32 doctors participated.

A scarcity of the new Salk poliomyelitis vaccine in 1955, and the "increased frenzy among the public" that resulted from that scarcity, offered the Society an opportunity to reach out to parents who were concerned about polio and their children. First and second graders were immunized in school, but the level of concern spawned by televised images of children in iron lungs created a demand far in excess of the supply. Dr. Amos Koontz drafted a press release to be published by the *Baltimore News Post*, advising parents that those most at risk, based on age, would be certain to receive the vaccine. The newspaper also included a form which could be completed and mailed in, should parents be seeking the vaccine but have no physician who could provide it, and the Society would help direct them to a source.

"Every parent quite naturally wants his child to receive the vaccine, and wants him or her to get the first available dose. In the urgency of their desire they are making it almost impossible for physicians, chiefly pediatricians, to practice medicine. Telephones in doctors' offices are ringing constantly, secretaries are unable to perform their other duties, and doctors themselves are spending unnecessary hours calming fears...and trying to keep down the mounting hysteria." The Society's press release went on to emphasize the danger of creating a black market for the vaccine, that "those who have pull or influence" may "get the first vials, those who have money to pay a premium get the second, and the devil take the hindmost." The Society laid out a plan by which those in the highest risk categories - children over one year of age, but not yet in the first grade - receive the vaccine before the upcoming poliomyelitis season.

The Society did learn to put the new medium of television to good use, however. In 1954 a series of weekly programs began appearing on WMAR TV. The first one, discussing arthritis, aired on November 5, 1955 and immediately drew the fire of several members. Two physicians were featured, and their names were given. Dissenters believed it to be more appropriate to call the presenters "Dr. X and Dr. Y," thereby eliminating any charges that the profession was cheapened by advertising. The Executive Board thought otherwise, and the programs continued throughout the decade, along with radio spots during Medical Education Week.

In order to reach even more citizens, in 1954 the Society created a Speakers' Bureau. Over a thousand local organizations, most of them churches, were contacted and presented with a list of topics on which a Society member would be willing to speak at an upcoming meeting. Within two weeks, the speakers' schedule was booked for ten months. Among the 31 topics were:

> "Arthritis - Forms and Fallacies"
> "Too Fat?"
> "How to Live With High Blood Pressure"
> "Why We Have Pre-Natal Care"
> "What Can Be Done About the Childless Couple?"
> "The Parent Problem and the Problem Parent"
> "Acne - Bane of Youth"

"Socialized Medicine"
"Oh, My Aching Back!"

Social events, from supplying coffee and doughnuts after regular meetings to staging more elaborate dinners and dances, occupied the Women's Auxiliary. The year 1956 closed with a Hawaiian Party for members and wives. The following March, the Auxiliary sponsored a dance at the Emerson Hotel after a regular meeting. The Emerson was owned by the inventor of the patent medicine Bromo Seltzer, a huge blue bottle of which in the memory of many present rotated slowly atop Bromo Seltzer Tower within a block of the University of Maryland (the bottle was actually removed in the 1930's). The evening's theme was the ocean cruise, replete with cruise fashions and a Captain's Table midnight supper. The year concluded when the doctors joined their wives for a party in the supper room at the MedChi headquarters on Cathedral Street. Dr Otto C. Phillips played Christmas music on the electric organ.

As the idyllic years of the 1950's came to a close there were few contentious issues to disturb the Society's agenda. The Women's Auxiliary continued to distribute the short film "Girl With A Lamp," created and underwritten by the Society to encourage young women to enter nursing. The Baltimore Regional Blood Center was opened in 1958 with the support of the Society. As membership grew the Society was faced with the need to hire secretarial help and find a larger space. MedChi, in financial difficulty throughout most the 1950's, raised the rent to $20,000 a year for what Dr. John De Hoff remembered as a "broom closet." Additional space was found with the state Faculty at its headquarters, negating the need for a physical move, and a rent reduction was also negotiated.

Membership stood at nearly 2,000 in 1959, up by 40% compared to a decade earlier. In a period in which accounts of meetings reflect a relatively calm environment in which to practice medicine in Baltimore (the exception being the continual, gradual incursion of government into medical decision-making, against which the Society had mounted a stringent and unwavering campaign), the summary offered by Dr. John N. "Jake" Classen, Secretary in 1959, was a radical departure. "In the past this report has been a statistical one, supposedly reflecting the growth and development of the organization. Such a report is, I believe, quite deficient," he wrote.

In the compact ten paragraphs which followed, Dr. Classen laid out a carefully worded plan for the future which called upon the Society to completely remake itself. "It has been apparent that the problems confronting the practice of medicine are mounting steadily...I cannot believe that the primary function of the Medical Society today is to stimulate research and be a media of postgraduate education," he proclaimed. He proposed major changes to the Preamble of the Constitution, so that the missions of the organization would become:

" 1) To protect the private practice of medicine against a welfare state.
2) To direct and mold any changes in this practice of medicine which might be prompted by the changing socio-economic standards.
3) To promote good public relations.
4) To protect and police our professional ranks.
5) To have an active grievance committee in whom authority is vested to take punitive action.
6) To negotiate contracts with Blue Shield, private insurance companies, and unions.
7) To set fair fee schedules.
8) To work in conjunction with the hospital councils to help the hospitals on matters of accreditation and education etc."

With this call to change the Society's function "from one of education to one of being primarily a medical union whose decisions might affect the autonomy and income of each and every member..." the Baltimore City Medical Society entered the tumultuous 1960's.

A New Role in Accreditation and Management

Yet as the decade dawned it appeared to be mostly business as normal. The proposed changes to the Constitution's Preamble were never voted upon. Dr. Everett S. Diggs, the new President, included nothing of the former Secretary's observations in his opening remarks, preferring instead to remind members that the parliamentary procedures outlined in Robert's Rules of Order will insure that the Society is able to maintain "a degree of control at meetings [that] is necessary in order to conduct the affairs effectively." The first major initiative was early in coming, and harkened back to the Secretary's fourth and eighth points, policing the ranks of medical practitioners and monitoring hospital quality control, hardly a revolutionary concept in the history of the Society.

Drs. Raymond V. Rangle and Joseph King presented a resolution to form a Baltimore City Medical Society Accreditation-Approval Monitor Board, the purpose of which would be hospital and physician accreditation. The Society's Charter gave it no authority in such matters without prior consultation with the state Faculty, and some members believed that this weakness created "an entering wedge for the corporate control of the practice of medicine." It was pointed out that the state Faculty already had such a committee, though there was no agreement among the members present on the effectiveness of the committee. One of the Resolution's sponsors, Dr. Rangle, noted that the state Faculty had thus far only handled grievances and not gone the next step to consider hospital accreditation. It was decided that an amended Resolution was necessary to delineate the role of the local Society more carefully as regards hospital accreditation and residency training.

Such a Resolution was drafted, which if approved would create a committee to act as a liaison between accreditation boards and local hospitals. The committee, however, was to be a function of the state Faculty, not the Society (a suggestion made by Dr. Amos Koontz). The Resolution was passed without debate by the Executive Committee and sent to the state organization. This conclusion was not unusual, as the city Society had often been the source of programs that would be better conducted on a statewide basis (1929 - rejection of a statewide anti-vivisection Bill, 1936 - appointment of "impartial physicians" as expert witnesses in state courts, 1938 - reorganization of the state coroner plan). In the early 1960's the Baltimore City group was still the preeminent organization in Maryland, as hospitals had not yet begun to move from the city to the surrounding suburbs.

Since its inception, the Society had played a major role in the establishment and governance of Baltimore area charity or city-run hospitals, in particular at Bayview and the Sydenham Hospital. The Baltimore Medical Association had been the first local organization to call for the establishment of a city-owned hospital for patients with contagious diseases. In 1921 the Society endorsed the plans of the Mayor's Hospital Commission to build a new hospital for the insane, and later lobbied for the expansion of that hospital. In 1960, the Society found it necessary to advocate against the provision of care for fee-paying patients at Baltimore City Hospitals, the newly-adopted name for the hospital at Bayview. Johns Hopkins University Medical School was at the time providing staff physicians and using the hospital to train medical students.

The controversy boiled over at several meetings, with the membership agreeing that the admission of elective patients, patients who could afford care in a private hospital, was against the mission of Baltimore City Hospitals and probably against the law. A letter to hospital management declared the Society's reason for its conclusion:

> "The basic controlling principle of the policy governing admissions is this statement - Baltimore City Hospital is owned, maintained, and operated by the City of Baltimore for the purpose of providing professional and hospital care for the indigent, or medically indigent, residents of Baltimore."

Hospital management was reluctant to tell the Society about the extent of hospital resources being used by private paying patients, but defended the right of City Hospitals to do so. While elective patients could, under the hospital's charter, be admitted for care, Maryland state law made it plain that such care could be provided only by registered physicians, not by medical students or unregistered hospital employees. Hospital management repeated that it would continue, even expand, access by private patients depending upon the educational demands.

There was at the time a proposal in City Hall to allocate in excess of three million dollars to the expansion of the facilities at City Hospitals, and the Society felt that an examination of practices there and perhaps a reorganization was necessary before it could be determined that this was a good use of taxpayers' money. While it was admitted that it was often difficult to find beds for the indigent - those who by the hospital's charter had first claim upon those beds - the extent to which private patients occupied those beds was not revealed by the hospital. Should taxpayers in effect supplement Johns Hopkins University by providing funding to expand educational opportunities for Hopkins students only at City Hospitals? The Society thought not, especially considering that the University of Maryland had no access to the facility and that "other segments of medical thought" were ignored by "the City Hospital's organization." "It was the consensus of opinion of the Executive Board [the Society's Board] that the main purpose of City Hospitals remains the care of the indigent." Clearly, the Society thought, City Hospitals had become "an exclusive facility of Johns Hopkins" and it was ignoring its mission of care for the city's poor. The April, 1961 Executive Board meeting closed with the appointment of a larger committee to study both the legal and medical implications of current City Hospital operations.

Apparently the University of Maryland was anxious to assume some of the staff responsibility at City Hospitals, and was angered that its crosstown rival, Johns Hopkins Hospital, had negotiated an exclusive staffing contract with the Welfare Advisory Board, the group that ostensibly oversaw hospital operations. The Baltimore City Medical Society adamantly supported the University of Maryland's position. Various staff members at City Hospital were referred to as "Hopkins men;" comments of those pro-Hopkins witnesses were deemed "provocative." The unspoken (at least at this point in time) objection of the Society was that privately-paying patients were being served in a hospital that had a closed-door policy to most Baltimore physicians.

By the end of 1961 a committee report was completed that called upon the management of City Hospital to do several things: First, remove the management from within the purview of the Department of Public Welfare, an inappropriate agency as the hospital would continue to make its resources available to private patients, and place it within the responsibility of the Department of Health. Second, immediately request that the University of Maryland make nominations to fill any existing vacancies in the Chiefs of Services at City Hospital. Finally, draw up a contract that will divide the management on an equal basis to be shared by both medical schools. Explicitly, Hopkins was to retain internal medicine, psychiatry, neurology and pathology, while the University of Maryland would manage general surgery, obstetrics, gynecology and radiology. In February of 1962 the agreement was drawn up by the Society and executed by every party. Baltimore City Hospital continued as an important teaching venue and its facilities were open to the majority of the city's practitioners.

However, the problem remained unsolved, as in 1966 City Hospitals again was accused by the Society of operating a closed facility. This time, the controversy exploded into a debate about whether ethical standards were being violated and led to a split between the Society and the state Faculty. The issue is covered in greater detail in the Medical Ethics Chapter, but suffice it to say here that in the end a new definition of ethical vs. unethical was crafted by the Faculty and each party left the ring bruised.

As if the split with the state Faculty over ethics issues was not enough, 1966 found the Society attempting to heal an internal rift that resulted in an insurgent slate being mounted for the first time in the Society's history. In the election of December, 1965, President-Elect Dr. Harry Connolly faced a challenger, Dr. Philip Wagley. Local newspapers branded Dr. Connolly as a "conservative," based on his opinion that the Society should honor a $50 surcharge on each member mandated by the Medical and Chirurgical Faculty.

The fee was to pay for advertising to fight Medicare. Dr. Connolly won by a slim, five-vote margin.

It was the $50 that riled members who were of the opinion that the Society should accept the fact that Medicare was going to become law no matter what they, the state Faculty or the AMA did, and figure out how to live with it. But the division had its real roots in an effort on the part of Dr. Connolly to unseat the current Society leadership, which he felt represented the interests of physicians from the city's two medical schools at the expense of the private practitioners. "The society cannot continue to exist with two opposing groups," he told a *Sun* reporter after his selection as President-Elect. Obviously, the call by outgoing President Dr. R. Carmichael Tilghman in 1962 had gone unheeded: "Let us welcome into our medical organizations practitioners and academicians on equal terms. Let us exchange the experiences in the ivory tower with those in the work-a-day world."

To contain the dispute, Dr. Connolly reached out to the insurgent members, and made efforts to assure that their perspectives would be adequately represented on the Society's many committees. "Town vs. Gown," "town" being the private practitioners and "gown" the academics, did not disappear entirely, but the two factions managed to conduct business in 1966. A year later, the boil settled down to a simmer, and when Dr. D. Frank Kaltreider was nominated as the next President-Elect he was unopposed. Virtually every other office that had a nominee from the supposedly bipartisan Nominating Committee was once again opposed by a member of the "liberal" wing, as it was described in local papers. The balloting, while featuring a more than normal number of write-in candidates, resulted in a balanced set of Officers and Directors. In 1967 the Society was able to settle down to normal business.

The year's first issue was another that had eluded a solution since telephones first intruded into doctors' offices. For years, the Society fought attempts by members to list their specialties in the yellow pages. Ophthalmologists had been particularly persistent, eventually earning the right to add "Practice Limited to Ophthalmology" next to their names. Of course, other specialists immediately adopted the same nomenclature and began pushing for a decision on whether the Chesapeake and Potomac Telephone Company could organize specialties into blocks, so that patients did not have to scan the entire alphabetical list of practitioners in search of, for example, a proctologist.

Throwing up its hands and falling back on earlier statements of policy, the Society agreed again to "reaffirm its previous position in regards to this matter. The action of the Board in 1961, and again in 1963 is reaffirmed as follows:

> "The Executive Board of the Baltimore City Medical Society feels that the phone book listing of physicians is an individual matter and does not feel the Society is involved. We do disapprove of any group listing as a specialty. Monitoring of the physicians so listed as to whether or not they are specialists is impossible."

Final word on yellow pages listings? Not exactly. In November, 1967, the Medical and Chirurgical Faculty stepped in with a statewide policy. Listings could be under one heading only: Physicians and Surgeons. Each listing could include only the doctor's name, address and phone number, an after-hours number and a home number. Listings describing the doctor's specialty, sub-specialty, or "Practice Limited to" were expressly forbidden. Display advertisements were out of the question.

The state Faculty was on a run, for in the same proclamation it instructed physicians that they must limit commercial advertising to "a personal, professional card no larger than three-and-a-half inches by two inches, upon which may be printed his name, title, address, specialty, telephone number, office hours and nothing else." Should a physician relocate his office, it was permissible to send notifications to his colleagues and his "bona-fide" patients as long as the notices were no larger than five inches by seven inches. It was deemed acceptable for a physician to hang signs on the building in which he practiced, but there could be no more than three of them and he or she should check with the Faculty first regarding the content of the sign.

Few of these agenda items harkened back to the 1959 message of Dr. John Classen, unless "Measles Immunization Sunday," the single day in 1967 when the Society vaccinated over 14,000 Baltimore youngsters, could be construed as recognition of the city's changing "socio-economic standards." Unless the dispute over yellow pages listings represented "policing the professional ranks," the Minutes of the Baltimore City Medical Society from 1960 through 1968 read like business as usual. Granted, the Society's protest of Medicare, though fruitless, did meet Dr. Classen's first objective: to protect the profession from the perceived adverse impacts of a welfare state.

But it was not until the Society's President in 1968, Dr. D. Frank Kaltreider, turned the gavel over to his successor accompanied in his farewell address by what was clearly a rebuke (the *Sun* called it a "tongue-lashing") to the membership, that the core missions of the Society were examined. "Our policy has been somewhat less than constructive where problems involving the health of the community have been concerned," Dr. Kaltreider said. He pointed to the cooperative committee that served as advisor in matters of health planning to the Regional Planning Council as an example of a constructive effort. "This is the type of positive activity that we should do more of."

Throughout the decade of the Sixties there were initiatives that took the focus from disease-specific discussions to topics of community health that represented more than just token reviews. In 1962, the state Faculty sent a resolution to the Society which, if passed, would demand "Full racial integration in all the health facilities and services of Baltimore and the State of Maryland." The Society voted boldly and affirmatively to support this resolution. Society President Dr. Houston Everett in 1964 served on a city-wide committee to study the increased need for outpatient services. Dr. Everett brought back to the Society a recommendation that it support expansion of not only traditional outpatient centers but also to include home care, in recognition of Baltimore's changing social and economic structure. From the Annual Report of that year: "Dr. Everett stated that with the passage of time, it was almost certain that additional calls will be made on our Society to participate in...social and economic problems," and that during the year the Society "experienced more than a flood tide of demand for economic and social change which many call progress, and although some of this so-called progress may be contrary to what many of us believe is for the best, much of it is good and that which is good deserves the active support and cooperation of organized medicine."

There were other indicators that the interests of Society members had changed, indicators that Dr. Kaltreider outlined in his last message to the Society as President. He announced then that the format of future meetings would address the social and economic problems arising from modern urban medicine. Two meetings, the historic first joint meeting with the Monumental City Medical Society, Baltimore's traditionally African-American group, on November 1, 1968, and the October 4 meeting that same year which resulted in a Memorandum committing Society resources to help in regional medical planning, had both been well-attended. "This is the type of meeting the physician in this city wants," he told the *Sun*.

Dr. Kaltreider was, however, correct in his assessment that much of the Society's time was spent in objecting, in casting negative opinions without offering positive alternatives, in failing to explore opportunities to "suggest constructive ideas." This course of action, he decided, "only encourages resentment, degrades the image of the Society and emphasizes a narrow acceptance of health problems. Offers of help and improvement are usually better received."

The Society's by-laws stated that the Past President automatically became the chair of the Nominating Committee. Dr. Kaltreider had several ideas suggesting how the Nominating Committee could reach more deeply into the membership for potential officers and committee members. The tradition was that potential officers and committee members were listed by the Nominating Committee and then these doctors were called to ask if they cared to serve. The result, Dr. Kaltreider believed, was that a large portion of the membership was left out of the process, to the detriment of the Society.

One of his suggestions was implemented in the next election cycle, when Dr. Kaltreider headed the Nominating Committee. A questionnaire was sent to every member, asking each if he or she had "any desire to use their talents in any of the offices of the Society or do they feel especially qualified to further the interest of the profession in any capacity?" Seventy-eight were returned. "I am not naive enough to believe that I will be deluged," Dr. Kaltreider admitted, "but if I can uncover one or two physicians whose talents can help the Baltimore City Medical Society, it will be worthwhile." Twenty of the nominees for the Annual Meeting at the end of 1969 were chosen from this list, twenty who undoubtedly would have not made it to the Nominating Committee's report had the old method been followed.

Another of his suggestions was designed to bring new members into the fold more quickly and maintain their interest. "A new member," he said, "should be asked what he believes the Society should be doing and in what areas he feels that he can contribute to its effectiveness as a voice for all segments of our profession." Current procedures enabled the 12-member Board of Directors to table a Resolution introduced by a member without submitting it to the entire membership. Dr. Kaltreider felt that this sent a message to new members that their input was unwanted. "A decision to kill a Resolution should be made at an open meeting," he advised.

The departing President did not limit his criticism to his own

Society. He was as concerned about the Society's effectiveness in matters pertaining to Baltimore City as he was the Society's influence statewide, which he believed was insufficient. In 1968, the Medical and Chirurgical Faculty had 3,140 active members, 1,541 of whom, 49%, were members of the Baltimore City group. In no case was Baltimore City represented in the state Faculty in a proportion representative of its membership. In the Council, 41% of members were from the City, and in the House of Delegates the city representatives amounted to just 38%. Also, the mechanism by which Council members were selected resulted in only a small percentage of those candidates recommended by the city Society actually being chosen to serve on the state Council. In most cases, the state Faculty rejected the nominees of the Society's Board and instead chose their own. Dr. Kaltreider suggested forming a committee to study the relationship of component societies to the state Faculty, with the goal of balancing the Society's representation and influence to match its membership and its contribution to medicine statewide. Such a committee was convened in 1969.

"With all the educational and practical experience in our power have we lost the ability to be constructive? Or can we only be against ideas?"
  -Dr. D. Frank Kaltreider

"Do you have any idea of the wide latitude of your responsibility under the law of professional responsibility? Do you understand fully the legal protection afforded by your membership in the Medical and Chirurgical Faculty and the necessity for financial coverage by an independent insurance company?"

-Letter from the Baltimore City Medical Society to its members
Unsigned
January 15, 1969 BCMS newsletter

"It is your Society. Show some interest in it!"
-from a letter to members of
the Baltimore City Medical Society
President Raymond C.V. Robinson, M.D.
February 12, 1969

"Every Physician will have to Become a Lobbyist"

Dr. Raymond C.V. Robinson gaveled the Baltimore City Medical Society into session on January 3, 1969, six years after his older brother, Dr. Harry N. Robinson, Jr., did the same upon becoming the Society's sixtieth President. "Metropolitan Medicine - Socio-Economic Aspects" was the opening topic for the year's first regular meeting, and a distinguished list of speakers was on hand. Dr. Robert E. Farber, the Baltimore City Health Commissioner, was joined by his counterpart in Baltimore County, Dr. Donald J. Roop and the Maryland State Health Commissioner, Dr. William J. Peeples. The session was "Acceptable for 2 hours Category I Credit by the American Academy of General Practice." The talk must have been compelling, for at the year's first meeting of the Board of Directors, two weeks later, the Board charged the Policy and Planning Committee to continue the study of the socio-economic situation in Baltimore City and make recommendations toward adapting the provision of health care to those changes.

Dr. Farber cemented a favorable relationship with the Baltimore City Medical Society that evening, which was confirmed by a letter from President Robinson to Mayor Thomas D'Alesandro urging that he reappoint Dr. Farber to the position of Commissioner of Health. "It is in the opinion of the Board of Directors of the Baltimore City Medical Society," he wrote, "that in these times of complicated metropolitan medicine...it would be unjust to the health of the population of Baltimore City to replace Dr. Farber and we strongly recommend his reappointment..." A *Sun* headline reported on January 13, 1969 "A Replacement of Dr. Farber Considered," and from a Florida vacation the Mayor commented that the city was "woefully weak in the area of health." A prominent attorney (not a physician), Francis X. Gallagher, was chosen by the Mayor to study the City's health needs. Earlier disagreements with the Mayor, especially regarding a Charter amendment that would move City Hospitals from a Commission affiliated with the Department of Health to the Welfare Department, affected City Hall's relationship with its Health Commissioner.

Mayor D'Alesandro was firmly of the opinion that the City needed to move from preventive programs like meat inspection to a proactive program to take health care direct to the citizenry. The opinions of the Society or Dr. Farber are not recorded in either the newspapers or meeting Minutes, and though the Health Commissioner agreed with the Mayor's plan to establish 20 local health centers, he worried about the "unnecessary burden to the department." Had this plan arisen a decade earlier there would have been an immediate objection filed by the Society, pointing to the participation of city government in health care as "socialized medicine." Dr. Kaltreider's late 1968 admonition, that the Society had better learn to accept what it could not change may have had the desired effect. Dr. Farber was reappointed to a six-year term.

Dr. Robinson's first official invitation to members announcing a general meeting topic opened with a bit of rhyme:

"Nothing but praise from the seriously ill,
The response to the Doctor's medical skill.
But woe to the Doctor's short-lived fame,
The recovered patient has put in a claim."

A panel of legal experts explained to the members the ramifications of potential malpractice suits, an issue that would remain on the Society's front burner for many years to come. "Tort Reform NOW!" was the refrain of nearly 1,500 physicians who marched at an Annapolis rally in January, 2004.

During 1969 the Committee on Public Medical Education maintained an ambitious schedule of television presentations. Weekly programs on WMAR (Channel 2) included discussions of alcoholism, glaucoma, marijuana abuse and cancer as well as general topics such as psychiatric disorders of the elderly and "The Family Practitioner of the Future." Members wrote the scripts and directed the shows.

Every month, each member of the Society found in his or her mailbox a printed announcement of the topics of coming meetings of not only the Medical Society but also its Sections, Study Committees, and the agendas of related organizations. From all appearances, the Society was a vibrant, relevant professional organization that had much to offer to its members. In March 1969, for example, the major topic was Cardiac Transplantation, with visiting speakers discussing patient selection criteria, surgical and immunological implications of the new surgery (Dr. Christian Barnard had done the first heart transplant in South Africa in December, 1967. Open heart surgery in the late 1960's was extremely rare). Topics of interest regarding professional liability insurance, office administration, third-party payment, efforts to reduce paperwork and tax issues for the private practice should have attracted new practitioners. Section meetings were geared toward issues of modern metropolitan medicine, including the treatment of alcoholism, the rising tide of heroin addiction in Baltimore, pacemakers, and the role of the psychiatrist in a modern city. Only after the more compelling subjects were discussed did the business meeting commence.

Yet general meetings were still sparsely attended, which prompted the letter from President Robinson in February, 1969 quoted in this chapter's title. The By-Laws were changed to require only 45 members present as a quorum (less than 3% of the total membership), but at the February General Meeting only 27 members remained in their chairs after the conclusion of the speaker's address. Dr. Robinson's letter was a sharp rebuke:

> "To those who complain that the Baltimore City Medical Society is controlled by an oligarchy, I reply that this is your own fault for not attending the meetings. In answer to your other complaints about meeting times and places and programs, most of you didn't even bother to answer the questionnaire stating your choices. When asked to serve on various committees, most of you refuse to participate."

The initial result was lengthy agendas for the March, 1969 meeting and an even longer agenda for the following Board of Directors Meeting. The situation made impossible Dr. Kaltreider's suggestion that votes on Resolutions be brought to the general membership rather than being settled by only the Board. Had the Society waited until "A decision to kill a Resolution [could] be made at an open meeting," nothing would have been accomplished.

There were important issues that would not wait for a quorum. Changes in the By-Laws of the Medical and Chirurgical Faculty threatened to reduce the representation of Baltimore City in its House of Delegates. Billing problems continued to arise with Blue Shield. There were countless accusations of overcharging and other cases of physician misfeasance. The vast majority of complaints were patient-physician misunderstandings and were amicably resolved, but they had to be dealt with all the same. The Board of Directors continued to conduct most of the Society's business.

Within five years, however, average attendance at a General Meeting rose to over 100. The decade began with a meeting at which no business could be conducted because of the lack of a quorum, and suggestions to correct the situation included having more out-of-town speakers or fewer meetings. At the end of 1970, however, the Policy and Planning Committee's report had some solid proposals: keep the new Peer Review Committee active, focus on socio-medical issues rather than socio-economic, work on building the proposed scholarship program. When Read's Drug Stores learned of a scholarship program, they asked if they could contribute to the fund rather than give physicians the usual Pikesville Rye and Whitman's Samplers. The Society said yes.

The January, 1971 meeting still had minimal attendance, but by May a committee had been formed to visit other urban medical societies to see what they did to bolster attendance and membership. The District of Columbia Society published a newsletter, had a lobbyist on retainer, and had a program available to support physicians' widows and help doctors with alcohol or drug problems. Philadelphia had successful orientation meetings, a large non-profit foundation, and five dinner meetings annually. A Baltimore City Medical Society newsletter began within months, and subjects for meeting presentations gradually changed. The Peer Review Committee found a chairman. A program to aid foreign-born physicians in Baltimore was begun, workshops for new physicians creating their first practices were instituted, and membership and attendance gradually improved.

Dr. John B. De Hoff, who was the Society's President in 1974, credited the improvement in attendance to the decision to address new topics at each meeting. He wrote in January of that year, "The criteria for medical society scientific programs are that the topics should be timely and pertinent to physicians, that they should be of value to physicians as individuals or as a society, and that they should interest a major part of the membership." In addition, he decreed that "To enrich the fellowship portion of the programs, coffee will be available before meetings and cold beer and colas will be added to the coffee and chocolate customarily served later."

The increase in attendance paralleled the rising awareness that private practitioners needed to pay more attention to the business side of their practices. Dr. Henry Wagner, President of the Society in 1980, recalled that "The Society took up 'business' issues as government and regulatory issues became prominent. It was no longer accepted that the medical profession by itself could maintain professional standards...Therefore the attention of the BCMS was directed toward government/profession interface." This is certainly reflected in the Minutes and newsletters of the period.

Other changes are noted, including the recognition of trends that the

Society had earlier either completely ignored or confronted negatively. In April, 1974, President John B. De Hoff, M.D. wrote that "BCMS was the first society in America to recognize that self-employed and salaried physicians have different needs for medical society services." Just twenty years earlier, the ethics of salaried physicians and their right to work as such was challenged in disputes over corporate and socialized medicine. Huge increases in those in the profession practicing specialties were observed and approved and specialists were no longer looked upon as threats to the general practitioner. The needs of immigrant physicians, minority physicians, younger physicians and physicians who worked in troubled urban settings were on the Society's agenda.

Throughout the balance of the decade of the 1970's the Society found itself faced with broader challenges and met them with new programs. Alternatives to the institutionalization of the elderly, genetic engineering, physician participation in the legislative process and freestanding centers for outpatient surgery were among the issues presented, and in 1976 incoming President Ian R. Anderson, M.D. was able to write that "The BCMS has been numerically the largest component [of MedChi] in the state for years...The BCMS ...has now become the largest in influence as well." The first professional lobbyist was hired in 1976. The Society was becoming a significant force in the political arena.

Richard Rombro, a Baltimore lawyer and later a distinguished Judge, accepted the post as BCMS lobbyist, and almost immediately jumped into the medical malpractice fray. Medical Mutual Liability Society, a physician-owned professional liability carrier, was created in 1974, and in 1975 Rombro and the Society reviewed a medical malpractice Bill to be introduced into the State Senate by Senator Harry "Soft Shoes" McGuirk. Both the Society and the state Faculty supported the Bill, which established a structure for mandatory arbitration of claims in excess of $5,000 and set the statute of limitations. During the 1976 session, lobbyist Rombro represented the Society in a total of ten legislative initiatives. The malpractice Bill was enacted, and the Society could report at the end of its lobbyist's first Annapolis session that "The medical profession has done very well in Annapolis this year."

The Society Grows into the 1970's

Growth in programs and members throughout the 1970's called for added staff and space. As early as 1968 the Committee for Policy and Planning brought a report to the Board of Directors suggesting that the time for a full-time Executive Director had arrived. The Board, however, concluded that "no lay person and no individual physician can substitute for increasing involvement and participation on the part of the membership" and nothing was done. Until then, the secretarial work had been accomplished by Mrs. Lucy McGuire, who worked for the state Faculty. At the close of the year, however, outgoing President Kaltreider subtly changed the title when he wrote that an Executive *Secretary* was needed. Bernadette Huber Lane, the Society's first full time employee was hired the following year and stayed for three decades.

A 1972 AMA survey suggested that the Society find a new, larger home, and in August, 1974 office space was found at the Village of Cross Keys. It proved to be a short-lived home, for new construction on a hill adjacent to the office resulted in periodic mud slides that found their way under the door and onto the floor of the offices. In just two years the need for a new home was recognized - this time to be purchased by the Society - and a Search Committee established to find the right building.

Perhaps the most important development of the 1970's was the creation of the Baltimore City Medical Society Foundation. A scholarship fund had been planned as early as 1971, but the discovery that the Society was in fact not a tax-deductible entity resulted in a 1972 Annual Meeting motion that was read and unanimously accepted: "The Baltimore City Medical Society should form a non-profit corporation which could accept tax-deductible contributions. Funds so received would be used for various educational and public health projects." Without that added attraction of tax deductibility, the growing financial needs of an expanding agenda could not be met. The Foundation's mission sounded compatibly like that of the Society as a whole: "to further stimulate research...enhance the quality of medical care...promote and preserve the public health..."

Within a month of the announcement of the formation of the Foundation in August, 1974, contributions started to trickle in. The first call for scholarship applicants went out in late 1975, seeking medical students who permanently resided in Baltimore to apply for financial assistance. The following year the first pair of scholarship recipients was chosen, and a total of $1,500 was granted. "The competition for the scholarship awards was keen," the newsletter reported in September. "The Foundation Board was gratified to find so many highly qualified medical school students from Baltimore City and had a difficult time making its decision." In 1977, five students shared a total of $4,000 in scholarships. Other grants established speakers' programs and financed the Alliance Against Venereal Disease's booth at the Baltimore City Fair.

THE BALTIMORE CITY MEDICAL SOCIETY - A History

The decade of discos and Vietnam ended when Mayor William Donald Schaefer declared December 6, 1979 as "Baltimore City Medical Society Day," to celebrate 75 years as a component society of the Medical and Chirurgical Faculty. The December Annual Meeting took place at Baltimore's Center Stage, with a buffet and champagne, and the production of *A Christmas Carol: Scrooge and Marley* rather than the usual educational session.

An ambitious list of new initiatives crowded the Society's agenda as Dr. Henry N. Wagner assumed the Presidency in 1980, foremost of which was the location of a proper downtown office. The Executive Committee spent all of 1980 searching. "With the renaissance of Baltimore City now well underway and the increasing availability of desirable real estate, we believe that we should increase our efforts to find a permanent home for the Baltimore City Medical Society," the March, 1980 *President's Viewpoint* declared.

While the search was ongoing, the Society's Legislative Committee was active, and opinions had radically changed. A second attempt was made to pass a Bill that would prohibit smoking in public places except those specially designated. (A 1964 Smoking and Health Committee motion to discourage the use of tobacco passed, but stopped short of insisting that hospitals' Women's Auxiliaries cease the habit of selling cigarettes to patients). The Society spoke out in favor of mandatory motorcycle helmet use. An important Bill would permit emergency medical technicians to legally provide care to a patient who was incapacitated enough to be unable to give informed consent (In the 1920's, the Society had resisted giving ambulance attendants permission to sever the umbilical cords in emergency deliveries, maintaining that only a doctor should do that). Support was given to a Bill that would increase the age for legal alcohol consumption. The Society had taken an activist role in the treatment of alcoholism already by "adopting" a Primary Alcohol Treatment Center a year earlier, and supporting it with volunteers and supplies.

Committee functions grew throughout the 1980's, and participation by members increased. There were programs that had been in operation for many years that continued, like the Boy Scout screening program at Broad Creek Camp in Harford County, which ended in 1985, not because of a lack of participation or need, but because of looming malpractice implications. Meeting attendance grew and credit was given to the Program Committee for devising a relevant and interesting series of speakers and talks. Dr. Raymond M. Curtis, for whom the Curtis National Hand Center at Union Memorial Hospital is named, spoke about his groundbreaking surgical techniques in 1980 and other prominent and respected practitioners were among the speakers who addressed the Society throughout the decade. Dr. Edmund Pellegrino, Director of the Kennedy Institute of Ethics spoke about "Ethical Aspects of Medicine: Who Lives, Who Dies, Who Decides" in 1989.

It was, however, the report of the "Baltimore City Primary Care Study" that was most awaited by the membership as the 1980's dawned. Conceived in 1978, the study's goal was to enumerate the amount of care provided to private patients by office-based physicians, as opposed to health maintenance organizations, community health centers, outpatient clinics and government health care operations. The data would be used to determine what adjustments in the types and levels of care were needed in the community. The Society allocated $10,000 toward the study, and employed a Hopkins graduate student to devise the method to collect data. Funding was sought, and received, from local foundations and agencies. It was obviously an aggressive effort on the part of the Society to improve health care delivery and solidify the role of the private practitioner in the mix.

The results of the two-year study were published in 1980 and revealed conditions which could have been anticipated, as well as some surprises. The mechanism to collect data was a questionnaire sent out by the Society to every licensed physician in the city. A phenomenal 90% of the questionnaires were returned. Much of the story that they told was encouraging. On average, Baltimore citizens were receiving more, and probably better, care than the national average. "Baltimore residents are receiving more preventive care services from more highly trained physicians than the national average," the study concluded. Half of the city's practitioners were affiliated with the city's two teaching hospitals, way above the national figure. The average amount of time a doctor spent with a patient was greater than that in other cities. Most of those physicians were still willing to accept new patients, suggesting that the availability of quality care had little to do with supply.

But discrepancies, largely geographic and economic, exposed weaknesses in the city's health care delivery system. None of these should have been startling, given the social environment of older east coast cities in general. Of course, the black population was underserved, and the physicians operating in poor black neighborhoods were underutilized. A black patient was only half as likely to go to a private doctor as a white patient in Baltimore. Medicaid made a difference, especially in the case of children, but not enough to even the demand for services across the city. The conclusion was that, even considering that black and poor patients were more likely to use ambulatory care from institutional providers (many of which were already stressed by patient volume to the point that care was degraded), improvements in delivery were imperative.

Increasing the number of primary care practitioners was not the answer, as office-based physicians had the ability to cover an additional half-million visits annually. Altering the mix of family practices and specialty practices could improve delivery, for it seemed that Baltimoreans visited general practitioners less than residents of other cities, and specialists more. Initially, the study suggested ways that the Baltimore City Medical Society could contribute to a re-adjustment of service availability and access:

"(a) Programs designed to recruit black physicians,
(b) Programs designed to recruit family practitioners, internists and pediatricians,
(c) Programs that would encourage the delivery of primary care by "intermediate" care specialists,
(d) Programs that would encourage the establishment of practices in the northeast, west and southeast districts of the city."

New Quarters on Park Avenue

Executive Director Bernadette Huber Lane recalled, in thinking about the years at Cross Keys during a 2004 interview, that "After one flood we had to renovate the entire office." "We had to move down the hall temporarily while they stripped the walls and floors." Running the Society while looking over her shoulder for the next mud slide became intolerable. Finally, in 1981, President Leon Kassel, M.D. could announce "I am pleased to have the privilege of announcing that the Baltimore City Medical Society has a permanent home." A former doctors' office, the red brick Italianate townhouse on Park Avenue was already undergoing renovation. The Board room would be in the stately parlour on the first floor, offices would occupy the remainder of that floor and the second floor, and the third floor could be rented. "The marble fireplaces were, unfortunately, both on the fourth floor," Executive Director Lane lamented. "I talked to the contractor - a great craftsman - about moving one of them to the Board Room, but it was embedded in the wall and would probably be broken in the attempt."

A sturdy brass plaque: "Baltimore City Medical Society - 819" was mounted on the brick next to the carved double front door, beneath an arched fanlight. The contractors with their brooms were just ahead of the movers, the painting having been completed just the night before the Society staff showed up with their typewriters and eight decades of records on November 3, 1981.

Just two days after the move, the regular meeting featured a mock interview by members of the Peer Review Committee that demonstrated that process and was followed up by a discussion of the problems with which the committee most frequently dealt and the outcomes of peer review actions.

Peer review had been a Society function as early as 1973. That year's report of the Peer Review Committee noted that it had examined 22 physicians - about 1% of the membership. "We feel that peer review, among other forces, is prodding us to keep pace with advances in knowledge without losing the will and wish to be physicians to the unwell." Most of the Peer Review referrals came from the Blue Shield Utilization Subcommittee, indicating that they had something to do with questionable bills. In one case, an internist was charged with making too many house calls. The newsletter's comment to that charge was "Would you believe it?". There were charges of ordering too many laboratory reports, too many procedures, and unnecessarily long hospital stays. The temptation is great to identify these as early examples of what commonly came to be called "defensive medicine."

Peer Review was an updated version of a standing committee with several decades of history by the time Lane and others wrote a new Peer Review Handbook in 1981. A Grievance Committee was in place years earlier, and dealt with both patient-practitioner disagreements and billing issues:

> "Dr. Connolly read a letter received from Dr....A letter will be sent to Dr....suggesting that the parties get together to work out an amicable solution to the complaint."
> -Baltimore City Medical Society Minutes,
> February 8, 1966

> "...a complaint was received by the Board from the Association of Insurance Adjustors that excessive fees were being charged by certain physicians...The Committee made an exhaustive study and discovered that some of the fees were outrageous...It was decided to invite one of the flagrant offenders to appear before the Board...The physician was contrite...and promised that he would mend his ways..."
> -Baltimore City Medical Society Minutes,
> December 4, 1959

In 1963, the name of the Grievance Committee was changed to the

Professional Relations Committee. This body was to deal with individual patient complaints, while the separate Peer Review Committee concerned itself with the overall quality of a physician's practice. Thereafter, a steady stream of complaints about billing practices, doctors' unwillingness to make house calls, and disputes between insurers and practitioners were addressed by the committees and reported to the Board of Directors. Grievance matters were not on the agendas of regular meetings, and the Minutes of Board meetings report only that a settlement was reached, that the matter was forwarded to the state Faculty Committee, or a decision was postponed awaiting the advice of counsel. The newsletter occasionally printed case histories, as a means of educating physicians how to avoid the communications problems that had already resulted in patient complaints. "In most cases, investigation revealed that the physician provided good medical care and his fee was appropriate. The vast majority of the complaints considered...are a result of poor communication between physician and patient," a 1986 summary of the committees' activities reported.

Peer Review typically resulted from a referral from the state Commission on Medical Discipline or from the Medical and Chirurgical Faculty. If the Society's Professional Relations Committee observed a trend in the complaints received about a single physician, or when the problems went beyond an individual grievance, action was taken. The process was involved, starting with a visit by committee members to the physician in his office, then an examination of patient records at the office and the hospitals at which the physician practiced. In nearly a third of the cases the Peer Review Committee handled, physicians had their licenses revoked or suspended, or they retired from practice. Another third resulted in a long period of re-education and follow-up conferences. The final third found physicians who were delivering an acceptable level of care, needing improvement only in minor areas.

It was the legislative arena which occupied most of the time and resources of the Society, however. In a 1983 speech to the American Society for Public Administrators, Executive Director Lane summed it up:

> "The Baltimore City Medical Society does not deliver health care; its individual members do, and they deliver most of the health care available in this community. A physician cannot practice without interfacing with the public sector. He is licensed by the state, must obtain a drug permit from both the State and Federal agencies, must have his office equipment calibrated in accordance with government standards, and receives an increasing part of his

income from publicly funded programs. Consequently, the medical society, as a representative of its members, must be involved with the public health care delivery system.

The Society's involvement begins in the legislature where policies are formulated into laws, and extends through the development of regulations for the administration of these laws..."

"This year, every physician will have to become a lobbyist," the January, 1985 newsletter announced. The Baltimore City Medical Society, if it had not done so before, with that statement set itself firmly on a course that its founders would have abjured. The final 20 years of its first century also found the Society advising its members that every physician had to become an insurance specialist, an attorney and an accountant as well. The Legislative Committee began 1985 by reviewing the host of medical cost containment initiatives that were scheduled to make their way to the floor of the historic Statehouse in Annapolis during the session. A 36-point report from the Governor's Task Force on Health Care Cost Containment was bound for the legislature. If passed, it would give broad authority to the Health Services Cost Review Commission (HSCRC) to set rates, determine which hospitals may offer what services and which may even be allowed to remain open. HSCRC could, if the Bill became law, mandate membership in Health Maintenance Organizations, and approve equipment purchases by physicians and ambulatory care facilities. It was the most sweeping set of medical practice regulations ever to have been proposed in a single legislative session.

In the State Senate, the Finance Committee was the first stop for the report, and the Society's relationship with power broker Senator Harry McGuirk was important. In the Maryland House of Delegates, the Environmental Matters Committee, headed by Larry Young of Baltimore City, was responsible for medical legislation. Richard Rombro continued to represent the Society as its lobbyist.

A dizzying array of 25 Bills passed under the Society's scrutiny before the session closed in early April; and the Legislative Committee published a list, including suggested stances each physician should take. The effects on the daily practice of medicine were potentially staggering: Physicians would have to apply for a Certificate of Need before purchasing selected equipment. Doctors would be required to advise their patients, in great detail, the amount covered by their insurance before providing care. The HSCRC would have the authority to set rates for services provided by physicians on hospital staffs. A state office would be established to act as a people's advocate, headed by an attorney. Hospitals would be required to submit data on individual physician performance without necessarily involving a physician in the interpretation of the data.

To the uninformed, it would have appeared as if the Society was opposing every measure ostensibly intended to insure that the best health care was provided at the most economical rate to the most citizens. Even the "Abortion - Prevention of Pain to the Fetus" Bill was opposed. The Bill failed to address the health of the mother, among other things. This, and other factors, led to the creation of an ad hoc committee to study the public's perception of physicians in general, and the picture it presented was not pretty. A Resolution was passed by the Society in March, 1985:

> "WHEREAS...a committee of the Baltimore City Medical Society has examined the public's perception of physicians and found that the public has a negative perception of the profession, and
>
> WHEREAS, this negative perception has been generated partly by unfavorable media reports...physicians may unwittingly be furthering this negative perception...
>
> WHEREAS, this negative public perception has an adverse effect on the Faculty's ability to achieve some of its purposes..."
>
> RESOLVED...a statewide task force be appointed...to improve relationships between individual patients and their physicians..."

That year, every physician was also called upon to become a public relations expert.

At the close of the 1985 session, the Society announced with obvious relief that "Legislation which would have been a step toward regulating where physicians practice and the fees they charge was defeated with the help of several key legislators...Now we must help them." The Baltimore City Medical Political Action Committee was a year old, and its primary purpose was to raise funds to assure that "legislators receptive to our views are elected." After a successful session, it was time for members to join the PAC and dig into their pockets to support the campaigns of friendly lawmakers.

Clearly, as Dr. Thomas E. Hunt, Jr. would later write in the February, 1993 *President's Comments*, "Politics is our Business."

"Whether we like it or not, politics is inescapable," he continued. The proceedings of the Baltimore City Medical Society, certainly since the 1985 pronouncement of each physician's new responsibility as a lobbyist, focused on the medical/political agenda at all levels of government. Medical malpractice issues rose to the fore again in the 1986 session of the Maryland legislature, and when Dr. Gary Rosenberg reviewed the year he noted that "1986 saw a dramatic rise in the number of Society members involved in legislative and political activities." The centerpiece of that year's work was the enactment of a $350,000 cap on non-economic awards in cases of medical liability, coupled with revisions of the law referring to evidentiary material, clamping down on the employment of "hired gun" witnesses by plaintiffs, and calling for a 10-year study of the effects of the legislation on the practice of medicine. "We hope that this first positive step in meaningful tort reform will encourage the reinsurance carriers to stay in the Maryland marketplace...relieving some upward pressure on premiums," President Rosenberg wrote at the session's conclusion.

It was not exactly a prophetic statement. Within a year Dr. Thomas Hunt reported that members were writing to their legislators urging the lowering of the statute of limitations and the limiting of double awards in the case of malpractice. Both Bills passed. Just one year later, in 1988, the legislature had before it a measure to control the rate classifications that Medical Mutual Liability, the Maryland physician-owned medical liability insurer, could establish for setting premiums. A measure was introduced which would have created a separate state agency, the Maryland Physician Liability Fund, into which doctors would be required to make deposits and from which claimants could be paid. Both measures were opposed by the medical community and both measures failed.

For the next two years the state legislature investigated other proposals that might have adversely affected a physician's practice and pocketbook. Included were the Health Services Cost Review Commission's privilege of setting physician fees, and the requirement that doctors advise their patients of the extent of their personal ownership of allied health care service providers. The goal of the latter would be, for example, to limit a doctor's ability to refer a patient to a lab owned in part by the doctor for tests, and to limit a physician's right to bill an HMO member if that physician is not under contract with that HMO. Tort reform and malpractice insurance were not on the radar screens in Annapolis.

As a striking indicator of the growing importance of professional organization in the face of dramatic change in the delivery of health care, incoming Society President Allan D. Jensen, M.D. opened his

January, 1992 column with the statement "Organized medicine continues to be our best hope to protect our patients' access to care, to preserve our traditions, and to address the problems facing medicine." He went on to cite a laundry list of challenges faced by the medical community, most of which could only be addressed by legislative action: managed care, increasing number of uninsured, reduced fee schedules, rationing, cost containment. "...all of these are concepts which are becoming increasingly familiar and burdensome and will make medicine more difficult to practice," he concluded.

Another challenge faced by the Society in turbulent times was the difficulty of maintaining a growing membership. Though the situation had not deteriorated so badly that it was impossible to do business because of a lack of a quorum, as was the case in the early 1970's, other forces intruded. The result was that many years after 1980 found more members retiring, moving themselves and/or their practices to the suburbs, or changing to non-dues paying status because of their age, than new members applying. This was, of course, nothing new. A century earlier the Baltimore Medical Association discussed combining forces with another society to boost membership, and debates over what would draw new members - more scientific sessions, fewer scientific sessions and more socio/economic sessions, opening the doors to "alternative" practitioners, social events after meetings, fewer meetings, - popped up sporadically.

Young Physicians Link Public Service to Membership

A June, 1990 retreat listed membership as one of four major areas of concern. One step taken immediately was the establishment of the Young Physicians Committee, under the guidance of Dr. John Ruth, which by February, 1991 had assembled three subcommittees and was searching for a public service project which would capture the imaginations of recent graduates. The intent was to draw new members from the large pool of new practitioners whose idealism had not yet been damaged by the reality of private practice in the HMO/Medicare/malpractice era. A Resolution was drafted in 1992 that outlined the public service project:

> "WHEREAS, the Public Service Subcommittee of the Young Physicians Committee has investigated the delivery of health care services to the homeless in Baltimore City and found that the care available is very limited, and
>
> WHEREAS, the members of the Baltimore City Medical Society are concerned about the lack of health care services

available...

> RESOLVED, that the members..support a program
> -to maintain and improve established sites where the homeless receive health care,
> -to provide a full range of medical services...from primary to subspecialty care...
> -to provide health education..."

The ambitious program called for volunteers to visit patients at Mayor's Stations, shelters and soup kitchens. A fundraiser was announced at the Senator Theatre, where the private screening rooms were rented to see "Far and Away" (starring Tom Cruise and Nicole Kidman) and five months later Dr. Ruth announced that 18 physicians had volunteered to work at shelters and another 12 had agreed to accept referrals from other homeless service agencies. Not only had a total of $7,000 been raised, but two retiring doctors had donated their entire examining rooms to the effort. Severe funding cuts suffered by the city's health department as well as drastic reductions in the Medicaid rolls made the work more important than the young doctors could have imagined when they set out.

Health Care for the Homeless, a local non-profit, experienced immediate increases in demand for their services. And the call went out for more volunteers. In 1992, 27 Society members volunteered their time, and nearly a hundred Society members were volunteering by mid-1993. The list of participating members included then Society President Dr. Thomas Hunt, as well as past Presidents Dr. Joseph Hooper, Dr. Hiroshi Nazakawa and Dr. Allan Jensen, and future BCMS Presidents, Drs. Donald Dembo, Konstantinos Dritsas, Jos Zebley, Willarda Edwards, and Beverly Collins. Over the first six months of the program, demand at Health Care for the Homeless doubled to over 230 patients per day. Most could not afford even the $5.00 co-pay required by the city's pharmaceutical assistance plan, and the Young Presidents Committee asked physicians to donate sample medications. The response was gratifying, but the demand greatly exceeded the supply. At the close of 1993, five Society members were honored for having contributed at least half-a-day a month at the clinic and cash contributions of $2,500 were given to Health Care for the Homeless.

Also in 1993, Executive Director Bernadette Huber Lane was honored as a Certified Association Executive, the highest accolade from the American Society of Association Executives. Ms. Lane had taken the helm of the organization 24 years earlier as Executive Secretary and maneuvered it through two difficult moves, first to the Village of Cross Keys and then to Park Avenue. "If Bernadette had not come to work for us, I don't know what would have become of the Society," Dr. John De Hoff commented in 2004.

The middle of the decade found membership and meeting attendance again in decline, repeating the cycle that had dogged local medical societies for over a century. More physicians were retiring from practice than entering the Society, and others were moving to the suburbs as hospitals did the same. By 1995, general meetings were attracting only 72 members on average, about half of the attendance 20 years earlier. Fewer than 10 new members were nominated monthly, whereas in 1973, the average monthly list of new members numbered 22. Joint meetings with the Monumental City Medical Society began years earlier, but now discussions began suggesting that the Baltimore County Medical Association and the Baltimore City Medical Society should hold joint meetings and combine their forces on particular projects. Some members thought that a complete merger ought to be considered. Both groups did gather in historic Westminster Hall in March for a presentation by the National Committee for Quality Assurance, a non-profit organization whose mission was to improve patient care through evaluation of health plans' quality control processes.

Out of that first joint meeting came a Joint Steering Committee. City members were appointed to the county's Committee on Managed Care, county members became active in the city's Public Information Committee. The societies agreed to combine efforts in the area of peer review, believing that by increasing the pool of reviewers a higher level of objectivity could be achieved.

The 1995 Maryland legislative session ended before the city and county committees could effectively join forces, but it was not without substantial victories for the medical community. "...as usual, BCMS physicians were the most responsive and spent the most time and energy in contacting legislators and getting their patients to sign petitions and call legislators," Executive Director Lane wrote at the end of the session. The highlight was passage of the Patient Access Act, which mandated that employers offering HMO plans must also include point of service plans as alternatives for their employees. Arrayed against BCMS, MedChi and the other local components was a deep-pocketed partnership of HMOs, Chambers of Commerce, insurance companies and industry, but the medical societies prevailed.

That same year saw the first Mini Internship, the brainchild of the Public Information Committee that had five city legislators shadowing physicians, doing rounds, seeing patients, filling out forms and reading reports for one day. At the dinner that followed, both politicians and physicians declared the day to be a success, and "admitted that there was much to learn from each other."

Dr. Murray A. Kalish, the first anesthesiologist to serve as Society President, began his tenure in 1996 by warning members that "Patient care will suffer if we as a society do not raise our voices in unison as the patient's advocate." He set three goals: Increase membership (it stood at 1,300 that year), expand the role of the new Managed Care Committee, under the chairmanship of Dr. Reed Winston, and explore anti-trust protection for physicians. Legislatively, the Society advocated in favor of handgun control and against weakening lead paint restrictions. The advocacy was successful, as was the Society's call for a statewide committee on HMO performance, for controlling an HMO's ability to limit the treatment alternatives a physician may offer to a patient, and to mandate that HMOs must make public the criteria used to decide contract renewals with care providers. "Physicians did very well in Annapolis," Dr. Gary Rosenberg, Chairman of the BCMS Political Action Committee said.

In spite of victories in Annapolis, successful new programs, and periodic joint meetings, membership numbers continued their decline. Dr. Kalish took every opportunity that presented itself to remind prospective members of the benefits to be derived from Society membership, but at the end of 1996 the Membership Committee could report only 30 new members for the year. Dues were reduced from $560.00, for both BCMS and MedChi membership, to $360.00. The 1997 legislative session again ended in victories for physicians and the Mini-Internships that year hosted five state legislators, two members of the press corps and two City Council members. After a May, 1997 message from President Donald Dembo, M.D. entitled "Apathy," however, the June meeting had to be canceled because of a paucity of registrants. The only highlight of the year was Physicians' Day in Annapolis, when 150 doctors went to the state capital to support their legislative agenda.

A questionnaire went to 600 members to determine if the Society was providing services that were pertinent to their needs. About a quarter were returned, and the message was that members understood the importance of legislative advocacy, were concerned that public education work to enhance the physician's image, and wanted their voices to be heard regarding contractual arrangements with managed care companies. A steering committee was appointed to mold the Society to the needs of its members. However, In 1997, only 28 new physicians joined the BCMS.

"Long cherished ways of doing things have to be revisited in the harsh cold light of declining physician autonomy, free time, and energy to devote to organized medicine," Doctors Jos Zebley of the City society and Ruben Ballesteros of the County group wrote in the September, 1998 newsletter. "Physicians question both our relevance to their experiences and their own ability to effect change in health care delivery systems." Combination of the two societies' functions was moving toward a complete merger. "Issues of combined governance, staffing, finding a common home for the combined society, dues structure (*we are shooting for less!*), all will need to be worked out in the months to come."

In the meantime, the Society worked to do more with less. Newsletter frequency was reduced from ten issues annually to six, and other mailings were curtailed. Dues again were reduced. "This is a gamble for the Society. We hope that we can make a...permanent dues reduction, but that will depend on how many new members join," Executive Director Lane wrote.

Ultimately, a complete merger with the Baltimore County Medical Association was rejected. "...many issues surfaced regarding the continued existence of a distinct Baltimore City organization to represent physicians and patients that work and live in the City," the Steering Committee concluded. The problems of drug abuse and violent crime, for example, were of more urgency to city members than county. In order to deal with the realities of declining membership, a problem not just for urban societies but for organized medicine nationwide, the BCMS chose to reorganize its structure, eliminate services that were redundant, and to consolidate services with other organizations.

While it was true that MedChi had made redundant some BCMS programs, some of these were originally the Society's, not the state Faculty's, initiatives. "Doctors Day in Annapolis," organized by Society Executive Director Bernadette Huber Lane, is an example.

Organizational Changes and a Corner Turned

"We are struggling," Beverly Collins, M.D., Society President in 1999, wrote. All local component Legislative Committees merged with MedChi's committee in 1999. The Baltimore County and Baltimore City societies created a consolidated Joint Managed Care Committee, and two of the general meetings every year were joint events sponsored by both organizations.

Plans to partner with the Monumental City Medical Society, Baltimore's affiliate of the National Medical Association, were underway, and many joint meetings resulted. Dr. James P.G. Flynn, chairperson of the Society's Continuing Medical Education agenda, was in discussions with the Baltimore County society and MedChi to pursue the joint sponsorship of the popular courses. A statewide movement toward consolidation was already underway, with the Anne Arundel County society planning to expand into Howard and Prince George's Counties, and the transfer of what were really statewide issues from other local components to MedChi, where they would more effectively be handled.

Executive Director Bernadette Huber Lane retired at the end of 1998, after 30 years' service to the Society. When Lisa B. Williams became the new Executive Director in March, 1999, she took the administrative helm of a group undergoing the most significant organizational change in its 95-year history. Williams brought academic credentials in social work and social welfare, coupled with a degree in law. She had extensive experience, both as a volunteer and staff member with various non-profit organizations and associations. Her legislative experience included work at the state level as a legislative liaison and a program specialist. All of her talents were needed to direct a leaner Society into its second century.

President John Manzari, M.D. reviewed the progress toward streamlining in the Summer, 2000 issue of the Newsletter. "We are planning to lease fully our Park Avenue building and relocate to the MedChi building on Cathedral Street," he announced. MedChi was to provide the required space rent-free for several years, but the Society withheld a decision to sell the Park Avenue headquarters until it could be determined if the arrangement was satisfactory. Two years earlier an attempt to sell the building was made, but there were no takers. Two-thirds of the building was already rented.

While the Society's patient-oriented newsletter, *BCMS Report*, was to continue publication on the existing schedule and format, the Society newsletter was reduced to one or two pages and members were encouraged to receive their issues by fax or e-mail to reduce printing and postage costs. Another questionnaire, to which only 16% of the membership responded, indicated that the activities among the two dozen offered by the BCMS considered important were the dissemination of local and state medical practice news, updates on legislation and regulation, representation in Annapolis and work to improve the profession's public image.

A buyer for the Park Avenue building stepped forward, and in April, 2001 the Society was relieved of the burden of a 130-year old rowhouse. The mini-internships went ahead with 3 state legislators, participation having been dampened by the September 11, 2001 terrorist attacks. The Society continued its ambitious program of

CPR training in Baltimore City public schools. Membership grew with 85 new names joining the BCMS roster, nearly triple the goal the Society set for itself at the beginning of the year. Five professional education programs were held that year, some in conjunction with the Monumental and the Baltimore County Medical Societies. At the end of the year, outgoing President Reed A. Winston, M.D. was able to report a successful continuation of educational and legislative programs, that volunteers, working with the Baltimore City Bar Association, had made important presentations on drug abuse in city schools, and that the Foundation had grown as the principal mechanism of public outreach.

September 11 left a mark on the agenda of Society regular meetings in the period immediately following the attacks. In May, 2002, Peter L. Beilenson, Commissioner of the Baltimore City Health Department, discussed "Bioterrorism: Responding to Patient Concerns." That same year. Dr. James P.G. Flynn, President of the Society that year, was appointed chairperson of Med Chi's Disaster Preparedness Task Force. An October special reception, on board the international hospital ship *Caribbean Mercy*, was well-attended according to Society Executive Director Lisa Williams.

Membership continued to be a challenge. Dues were reduced to $195.00, statewide, for all first-time members. When the Membership Committee wrapped up 2002, it could report some good news, as the retention of freshman members was high.

New Membership, New Leadership

Dr. Eve J. Higginbotham took the helm of a leaner organization in 2003. The title of the *President's Comments* in the March issue of the BCMS newsletter, "History Repeats," was appropriate as the Society prepared to celebrate its 100th anniversary. She listed among the problems faced by professional caregivers the rise of IIIV infection, the growing difficulty in collecting bills, the problem of delivering care to the uninsured, and the ongoing effect that Medicare and other governmental initiatives were having on the practice of medicine. "Yes, the more things change, the more they remain the same," she concluded.

This is a sentiment that has arisen frequently in the preparation of this celebration of an important and effective professional organization. But it is not entirely accurate. Dr. Anil Uberoi assumed the Presidency of the Baltimore City Medical Society in 2004 at a well-attended meeting in Baltimore's Inner Harbor. She was the first physician of East Indian descent to rise to that position. In accepting the office, Dr. Uberoi addressed an audience that would have amazed the physicians who gathered on North Eutaw Street a century earlier. Dr. Henry Ottrage Reik, who chaired the committee that created the Society in 1904, would not have seen an African American face as he scanned his colleagues around the table. Nor would he have seen a woman, not even the spouses of the physicians present, though women had been among the students at Johns Hopkins since 1893. In the crowd at Dr. Uberoi's investiture were a number of women wearing their native saris. Foreign-born physicians in the 1904 organization would have been limited to those from western European nations only.

After Dr. Eve Higginbotham turned the gavel over to Dr. Uberoi and the guests completed their international meal, a jazz band opened its first set. There was no tobacco smoke clouding the room. Between numbers there was no talk about yellow fever or smallpox. The water in the pitchers on every table was safe to drink - straight from the tap. The gutters outside the Harbor Court Hotel were not filled with raw sewage. If the gaiety of the evening were disturbed by the sound of a siren on Light Street, it may well have been atop a Baltimore City ambulance dispatched from the fire department adjacent to the Bromo Seltzer Tower. Among the sponsors of Dr. Uberoi's induction was a pharmaceutical company and an insurance company, an indication of the improvement in the relationships among physicians and these two important members of the wider medical community.

"We have, as a membership organization, turned a corner," Executive Director Williams said in 2004. Membership was on the rise, with 117 new members recorded in 2003. "Physicians' one-on-one contact with their colleagues is the key to building a bottom-up membership organization," Williams commented. Recent events strengthened efforts to increase participation. A January, 2004 rally in Annapolis to demonstrate for tort reform sparked interest in professional organizations. As a follow-up to two retreats in 2003, the Board began developing a strategic plan to better focus on membership and other priorities. "The Board's focus is much larger now," Williams noted, "and they are more engaged."

Programs were attracting greater interest as well. The popular Mini-Internships, in which a layperson accompanied a physician for a day in his normal duties, were on track. "A Day with a Doc" attracted businesspeople and leaders of organizations, largely because of a partnership between the Society and the Greater Baltimore Committee. Baltimore City Public Schools and CareFirst expressed interest in participating in an outreach program to address the problem of childhood and adolescent obesity.

Things do change. The centennial of any organization is a time to look back, and in doing so it becomes difficult to agree with Dr. Frank Kaltreider's 1968 characterization of the Society as a reactionary, negative force. Throughout its history, as well as the histories of the groups that came before, professional medical organizations have served both their physician members and the community at large admirably, especially given the complex nature of modern medicine.

"Most of us have become physicians because of our desire to help patients, and for the intellectual satisfaction involved. Despite economic and political changes, medicine continues to be among the finest and noblest of professions, and we must be careful not to dissuade future generations...The new generation should be encouraged to accept the challenge of medicine, to work for the betterment of their patients and society."
-Allan D. Jensen, M.D.
President's Comments, August, 1992

"The Board of Censors regrets that we find it necessary to report at this time an ever increasing dissatisfaction among the members of our fraternity...there is a progressive tendency to disregard that courtesy among physicians which has been characteristic of the medical profession.

This disregard of the principles of medical ethics is not confined to the men recently admitted to our ranks...but it is charged more especially against those, who by their position should be our leaders and whose ethical conduct should set an example to the younger men...

While the Board of Censors is not in a position to take up the investigation of such charges...it is incumbent upon us to sound a note of warning."

-Minutes of the Baltimore City Medical Society
April 7, 1908

"WHEREAS, It appears to the General Assembly of Maryland that the establishment and incorporation of a Medical and Chirurgical Faculty or Society of Physicians in this State...may in future prevent the citizens thereof from risking their lives in the hands of ignorant practitioners or pretenders to the healing art;"

-Preamble to the 1799 act
of the Maryland General Assembly
which created the
Medical and Chirurgical Faculty of Maryland

Medical Ethics

When the Baltimore City Medical Society's Board of Censors dictated its April, 1908 report chastising some of its members for "infractions of the Code, which are constantly poured into our ears," the ethical breach that sparked its creation addressed the relationship between general practitioners and specialists. The role of the family physician was assiduously protected by the Society's code, and allegations that specialists "dropped the regular attendant from the case, without ceremony," or worse, recommended the patient to a friend or associate who happened to be a family doctor, were viewed as serious ethical transgressions.

It was a concern for the ethical practices of health care professionals that spawned the first professional organizations both locally and nationally. Constitutions and mission statements are replete with language such as "dignity of the profession," "maintenance of etiquette," and "elevate professional standards." Off the record, early members of medical societies were more likely to refer to "villainous quacks" when discussing the medical ethics as a reason to organize. (The original use of the word "quack" was to describe a person illicitly posing as a doctor, though in modern usage it is more likely used to defame, in the opinion of the speaker, a bad doctor. It is actually an abbreviation of an early English term, "quacksalver," used to brand anyone who quacked like a duck about the virtues of his salves.)

Baltimore's first local medical society was founded expressly for the purpose of putting an end to the ministrations of untrained practitioners. Dr. Elisha Hall, of Frederick, Maryland, expounded on the wisdom of creating a "medical establishment" that would nominate three physicians to examine and license all applicants to the practice of medicine. Dr. Hall was a colleague of Dr. Charles Frederick Wiesenthal, who was instrumental in establishing the first Baltimore medical society (1788), and was active in that organization's earliest days. His proposed plan for examining physicians called for even established practitioners to stand for examination, because "we are surrounded by swarms of quacks."

The 1788 society was an abortive attempt, and before a local organization could become firmly established the state Faculty was organized. The first meeting of the Maryland Medical and Chirurgical Faculty took place in Annapolis on June 3, 1799. Baltimore's, and the state's, most eminent physicians were present: From Baltimore City, Dr. George Buchanan, the only Baltimore doctor bold enough to sign his name to letters to the editor regarding the failed local Society of a decade earlier, and Dr. Ashton Alexander, who lived until 1855 and was instrumental in establishing other Baltimore City organizations. Others who gathered near State Circle included Dr. William Beanes, of Potomac, whose capture 15 years later by the British Army led to the writing of *The Star-Spangled Banner* by Francis Scott Key.

Dr. Alexander was the only Baltimorean chosen to serve on the Faculty's first Board of Examiners, the committee charged with the responsibility of judging the skill of each applicant for a license to practice medicine in the state. Dr. Alexander was familiar with the extraordinary level of incompetence among those claiming to be medical doctors. A colleague of Dr. Andrew Wiesenthal, Dr. Alexander assuredly shared the younger Wiesenthal's opinion that "in physic in this part of the world the most errant quack, if he has assurance enough, will often claim the preference and obtain it before a man of real and true abilities."

With the founding of the American Medical Association in 1847, a national Code of Ethics was published that eventually became either the model for state and local codes or was adopted by those groups wholesale. But even before the AMA, a Baltimore group painstakingly wrote its own code, much of which it later claimed was used by the new national organization. The Medico-Surgical Society of Baltimore, under the leadership of Dr. Samuel Baker, spent much of 1832 on the project. The Minutes which survive indicate that 100 copies of the code were printed and distributed to the members in August of that year. The next year the creation of a Fee Bill was proposed, an attempt to standardize physicians' charges and thus lend credibility to the profession. Neither the Code of Ethics nor the Fee Table survives.

Though often referring to the AMA code, Baltimore societies were left to grapple with local issues of medical ethics throughout their history. The Baltimore Medical Association worked in partnership with the Baltimore Pathological Society in 1873 to clarify several ethical questions, in particular the problems of specialist and physician advertising. The Association chose to accept the Pathological Society's proposals which stated that specialists should be required to uphold the same standard of ethics as general practitioners, including a ban on advertising. Members of the Association were forbidden to refer cases to specialists who violated the code. Curiously, the Baltimore Pathological Society closed its doors less than a year later after one of its leaders was convicted of medical misconduct.

Eventually, most considerations of ethical points devolved to three principal questions: Did an applicant for membership in the Baltimore City Medical Society practice any form of "sectarian" medicine (defined as something beyond the normal, university-taught methodology)? Did a physician maintain a relationship with a druggist, own a drug store, lend his or her name to a maker of patent medicines or in some other way profit by the sale of proprietary medicines? Did a physician engage in any other "commercial" activities beneath the dignity of the profession?

Sectarian medicine proved to be the issue that could not easily be put to rest, especially as it applied to homeopathic and osteopathic physicians. Homeopathy was widely practiced in Baltimore. The first homeopathic practitioner in the state hung out his shingle in southern Maryland in 1833. By the Civil War, homeopathy was the preferred medical care of many of Baltimore's wealthiest citizens.

The AMA ultimately gave up on trying to reach at a decision about homeopathy that satisfied its members. When the problem of the recognition of homeopathic physicians first arose in 1870, the Committee on Ethics called the practice "cult medicine," and determined that it was plainly in violation of the Code of Ethics. The New York (City) Medical Society subsequently loosened its strictures on homeopathy, and for its progressiveness was expelled from the AMA A newly formed allopathic group, the New York State Society, was granted admission, and in 1903 the national Association threw up its hands and instructed each state and local agency to arrive at its own guidelines regarding sectarian practice.

Thus the Baltimore City Medical Society was faced with what appeared to be an intractable problem in its very earliest years. At the semi-annual meeting in April, 1906, the Board of Censors brought the topic of admission of homeopaths to the floor.

"According to the By-Laws of our Society, every reputable and legally qualified physician in Baltimore is eligible, who does not support, or practise, or claim to practise sectarian medicine. And this ruling debars all those who are ostensibly practising homeopathy, and those who are connected or affiliated with homeopathic colleges, hospitals and societies." The question arose after several members of the homeopathic community expressed interest in joining the Society.

One of the applicants was Dr. O. Edward Janney, mentioned briefly earlier. His case is worth examining because it is an example of what made the problem so perplexing to the Society. Though a devoted homeopath, Dr. Janney was also a registered pharmacist and a graduate of the University of Maryland School of Medicine, class of 1881. He was well known and respected in the Baltimore medical community. That, plus a member's recommendation, was typically all that was required for membership in the Baltimore City Medical Society. Dr. Randolph Winslow, a faculty member of the University of Maryland and a past Vice President of the state Faculty, recommended Dr. Janney as a desirable member. Dr. Charles O'Donovan, Jr., who attended medical school with Dr. Janney, decreed him "a man above reproach."

"A letter was read from Dr. Gundry in which he stated that due to happenings of recent years on the Homeopathic Board we should not accept their licensures for membership in this Society"
-Minutes of the Baltimore City Medical Society
March 27, 1956

To understand the appeal of homeopathy in Baltimore and elsewhere it is wise to recall the situation of allopathic care when homeopathy first arrived on these shores. Dr. Benjamin Rush, the most respected physician of his era, routinely bled patients until they were "as white as veal" and treated them with huge doses of mercury. The countryside was littered with practitioners who alternated from blacksmithing to farming to "doctoring." Faith in the medical profession in the early 1800's required a strong will.

Other alternative medical practices also flourished, in particular the herbal remedies of the Thompsonians. By 1838 the influence of Thompsonian practitioners in Baltimore had grown so that they were able to have the Maryland State Medical Board closed, allowing anyone - with or without any credentials at all - to practice medicine.

After he purchased a copy of *Hering's Domestic Physician* at a Baltimore bookstore in 1837, Dr. Felix McManus opened an early homeopathic practice in Baltimore City. The appeal of homeopathy grew rapidly, and several societies were created to serve the same function as allopathic organizations. There was an abundance of infighting among competing groups, even after the founding of the Southern Homeopathic Medical College and Hospital of Baltimore in 1890. An earlier group had opened the Baltimore Free Homeopathic Dispensary in 1878, and there was a bitter debate about how to treat paying vs. indigent patients (traditional practitioners were struggling with the same issue). The City of Baltimore recognized the hospital, giving it badly needed credibility, by providing $800 annually beginning in 1895, when the school adopted a 4-year curriculum. The state eventually provided $5000 each year in support.

Further recognition came when, in 1892, the State of Maryland re-established the State Medical Boards, in the process creating two bodies, one for traditional medicine and another for homeopathy. But strife among the various practitioners continued to degrade the practice in spite of government support. The Great Fire of 1904 indirectly destroyed the Southern Homeopathic College, not by burning it down, but by cutting off state support which went instead to the rebuilding of the financial district. In addition, other groups of homeopaths created two new institutions, the St. Louis Homeopathic Hospital and the Maryland Homeopathic Hospital. The old Southern Homeopathic College became the Maryland Medical College, an allopathic school admitting students who were unable to get into other universities. After receiving a terrible review in the Flexner Report of 1910, a study of all 131 medical schools in America and Canada enthusiastically supported by the AMA, the Maryland Medical College closed. In 1912 the Federation of State Medical Boards was founded, and accepted the AMA's evaluation of medical schools, spelling the end for schools that taught alternative medicine. By 1921 there were no homeopathic institutions left in Baltimore.

The state Homeopathic Board continued in existence despite the decline in practitioners, and in 1956 the Baltimore City Medical Society faced the issue of admitting homeopaths for the final time. Dr. Joseph Kwei Yuan, who served on the Board and was also on the staff at Doctor's Hospital, applied for membership. Because he was a hospital staff member, the Society could not turn him down, and chose instead to grant associate membership. Dr. Yuan sent in a $60 dues payment, which was for members with full privileges, and the Society wrote to the State Board of Medical Examiners for a decision on whether "they believe that people approved for the Homeopathic Board are fit for membership." Dr. Yuan was ultimately granted associate membership only.

The discussion continued. It happened that Dr. R.E. Cabot of Boston was in the audience, and he outlined the actions taken in Boston toward homeopaths. He stated that "the bars have been let down, but that homeopaths were obliged to pass the same State Board examination as regular physicians." Dr. Samuel T. Earle reminded the members that while president of the state Faculty he had mounted a fight in favor of admitting homeopaths who were otherwise qualified, and his opinion had not changed.

On the other side of the aisle, Dr. James Rowland, a member of the Board of Censors, put himself on record as opposing the admission.

While "personally having nothing against Dr. Janney," he urged the Society to interpret strictly the clause in its by-laws against sectarian medicine. Dr. Charles E. Brack, Chairman of the Board, was anxious for a decisive vote. "Dr. O.E. Janney is not fully endorsed by the Board," he stated, "but is presented to the Society so that the momentous question of admitting homeopathic physicians can be determined by general vote and a precedent established...The Board fully appreciates the personal qualities of Dr. Janney and is favorably inclined to Dr. Janney's admission, but as any action would mean to either open or shut the door, we prefer to have the Society make its own decision."

Finally, Dr. Earle moved that the report of the Board of Censors be accepted and that a ballot be taken regarding the acceptance or rejection of all of the candidates, Dr. Janney included. This was done, and every candidate, including the homeopath, was admitted. The exercise, in addition to the fact that it did not set the final precedent for which Dr. Brack had hoped, was academic. The following year, Dr. Janney, also a dedicated Quaker, retired from his medical practice to devote himself to social causes. He was active not only in seeking the rights of women to vote, but also in campaigns to end "white slavery," or forced prostitution.

Two years elapsed before Dr. Brack was again forced to bring the matter to the general membership. In December, 1908, the Board of Censors returned with the news that two of the Society's members were in fact serving on the Homeopathic Review Board. One, a Dr. Garrison, transferred to the Baltimore City Medical Society from a surrounding county. He submitted his resignation and it was accepted. The other, Dr. Bowman Hood, was not affiliated with a homeopathic institution when he became a member of the Society, but his acceptance of a position on the Homeopathic Examining Board put him squarely in violation of the rules. Apparently, he was not as accommodating as Dr. Garrison and did not resign. The Board laid the decision at the feet of the general membership, repeating that it would refuse applications from those practicing any form of sectarian medicine "unless the society decides to repeal that portion of the by-laws, which refers to this class of practitioners."

That meeting closed without a decision on the matter, leaving Dr. Brack and the Board of Censors again to strictly follow the by-laws regarding the eligibility of homeopathic physicians. But before adjournment there were several other ethical problems on the table. The first concerned an accusation made by one member that another had "defamed the character" of the complainant, and that a suit against the alleged defamer had been brought asking damages of $10,000. The Board of Censors, having already met with the two parties' attorneys, was able to tell the members present that "After carefully weighing the evidence presented, the Board decided unanimously that the charges were not sustained." The Society was also told that another of its members had been convicted of illegally selling cocaine, and that member was summarily dismissed.

The conundrum of recognizing practitioners of alternative forms of medicine proved resistant to the Society's or the Faculty's efforts to purge the medical community of what was considered questionable practice. House Bill 413, introduced into the Maryland General Assembly's proceedings in 1927, would have given a green light to osteopaths, with little regard to training or qualifications, to perform surgery and prescribe drugs. The Bill was so vague that in spite of the claim "that there does not exist in this state an osteopathic surgeon or an osteopathic physician who is qualified to practice surgery or prescribe drugs," no limitations on the practice were outlined. The Society objected vehemently, and Delegate Ensor withdrew his legislation.

Various other individual cases arose as one Baltimore physician or another was convicted of a civil or criminal transgression. Equally unethical in the eyes of the Society was "commercialism," which in a previous meeting had been declared by Dr. Brack to be "lowering the standards of the profession." When Dr. Wilmer Brinton spoke out, observing that "some of the members appear to have press agents," no action was taken but a number of heads must have shaken in disbelief. That April, 1908 meeting closed with the recommendation by Dr. Brack that principles of medical ethics ought to be taught in colleges.

Politics and Medical Ethics

For over two decades, before and just following World War II, the Baltimore City Medical Society's schedule was filled with discussions on insurance, public health and eventually war. The clinical presentations continued unabated, though the agenda was altered to put these talks at the beginning of each evening meeting, due to "the propensity of members to leave early." Ethical issues slipped to the back burner.

This ended when Dr. Amos R. Koontz assumed the Chairmanship of the Committee on Public Medical Education in 1949. Beginning the following year, Dr. Koontz led the Committee and the Society into the maelstrom of McCarthy-era politics, when he called for the Society to "apply for a place on the Coordinating Council of the Maryland Committee for Representative Government," the state equivalent of the Congressional committee from which Senator Joseph McCarthy investigated alleged communist infiltration. A unanimous affirmative vote was followed by acceptance of Dr. Koontz's proposal to endorse the agenda of the Maryland Committee Against Un-American Activities. At the Annual Meeting in 1950, the Committee was "commended for the work that it has done." The work mixed both issues of medical ethics and the threat of government-mandated medical insurance, blurring the lines by suggesting that a supporter of any government plan, anyone brought up before the House or Senate Committees on Un-American Activities, or anyone expressing an opinion to the "left" of the Committee on Public Medical Education was in fact acting against the accepted rules of medical ethics. Ultimately, it would go so far as to investigate whether a white doctor who sold his house to a black family ought to be allowed to continue practicing medicine.

Under Dr. Koontz, the Committee on Public Medical Education became a mechanism for propagandizing against "socialized medicine," which translated into any form of mandatory medical coverage that would include payments to individual practitioners. Dr. Koontz also used the Committee as a tool to support the efforts of the conservative McCarthy Committee on Capitol Hill to root every element of "socialism" and "communism" out of American society. Some of the initiatives, notably the publication of the comic book *The Sad Case of Waiting Room Willie*, proved to be embarrassments to the Society, especially after McCarthy's demise.

"While this story of 'Waiting Room Willie' has been portrayed humorously, he is real......Because everything that happens to Willie has actually happened to REAL people now living in countries that have tried or are trying the same type of government-controlled medical care now proposed for AMERICA!"
-from *The Sad Case of Waiting Room Willie*
Baltimore City Medical Society

Thus begins the comic book chronicle of *The Sad Case of Waiting Room Willie*. Congress has passed a National Health Insurance law and the hapless Willie is taken sick at the factory where he works. One of his cohorts suggests "Whyn'tcha go get some of that FREE medicine?" Willie pulls his hat down over his bowl haircut (reminiscent of Shemp, of "The Three Stooges"), punches out, raises his umbrella and steps out onto a rainy Baltimore street. He heads to the office of "Ol' Doc Jones...He's just like a relative, knows me like a book..."

But upon entering Dr. Jones's waiting room, Willie encounters a long line of restless patients. Dr. Jones's nurse sympathizes, but Willie has not registered on the doctor's "panel." To treat Willie, even if he were able to wait in the long line, might cost Dr. Jones his license. "Here, Willie," the nurse pats him comfortingly on his shoulder, "Go see Dr. Smith, I hear HIS panel isn't quite filled and you do look rather sick..."

So Willie starts a long and torturous odyssey, encountering lines of fur-wearing patients who are there because it's free and because "I just love going to doctors...gives me someone to talk to." He labors through the dreaded "triplicate forms" and is accosted by a gentleman with a fake moustache, selling bootleg aspirin from a trash can. "It'll take you THREE DAYS and two TRIPLICATE forms to fill out before you get it...you may be dead by then." After collapsing in the street, poor Willie is carried to the General Emergency Hospital in a police van where he gets about 10 seconds of a doctor's attention. "No time to have a lengthy talk, friend...got 43 more emergencies!" Willie's mother rushes to "Doc Rural's General Store," only to find that the doctor has abandoned medicine and is running a confectionary. "I didn't study ten years to be a political job-holder and take orders from some ward-heeler," he proclaims. Finally, after having his appendix removed on his kitchen table by "Ol' Doc Jones," Willie decides that he will write to the guy "holdin' down a FAT job with the GOVERNMENT" to complain. "Looks like Medicine's gone back FIFTY YEARS!," Dr. Jones exclaims as he rolls down his shirt sleeves.

In its publicity for the 16-page comic, the Society called its publication "...a collection of incidents, most of them from factual reports of occurances [sic] under socialized medical plans in other countries, but all happening to one poor waif, who is really sick and unable to get medical care under the New Utopia..." Physicians were asked to purchase 250 copies each ("less than the cost of a subscription to Time, Life, etc. to be found in most waiting rooms"). The Woman's Auxiliary helped with distribution, and *Willie* appeared on Baltimore news stands for a nickel.

Despite its simplicity, condescending attitude and its disregard of the actual proposal from the White House, *Willie* received flattering reviews. "The Baltimore City Society is to be complimented on its enterprise in using comic book techniques to tell the story of Socialized Medicine," wrote the Medical Society of the County of New York. "Not very dignified, perhaps, as a Medical Publication, based completely on the psychology of ridicule, but very readable, amusing and carried its points well...certainly would have great appeal to the boys sipping in the barrooms, in barber shops...And if and when votes for Socialized Medicine are counted, the crosses those boys make on their ballots count just as much as anyone else's vote," gushed the Maryland Commissioner of Mental Hygiene Dr. Clifton T. Perkins.

Five years after the printing of 12,400 copies of "Little Willie", 500 remained in inventory. Dr. Robert Kimberly, Society treasurer, called the comic "the bad product of the Committee on Public Medical Education." The members present at the February 19, 1957 meeting unanimously voted to dispose of the balance.

But until "Little Willie," the Committee on Public Medical Education was one of the Society's dominant forces. Dr. Koontz wrote in his 1950 annual report that "I shall make no attempt to give a detailed account of the many meetings we have held, of the public addresses, radio talks, television appearances, letters written, articles published, etc. Suffice it to say that your Committee has been very active along these lines." In his weekly *Sun* column, Louis Azrael reported on January 23, 1951, that newly-elected Baltimore City Medical Society President Dr. Louis M. Krause had opened a meeting with a prayer. "The assembled doctors were shocked," Azrael wrote. "It was the first time in the long history of the medical association that any such thing had happened."

In Dr. Krause, Dr. Koontz had a partner with whom he shared similar political sentiments. Under the anti-socialized medicine banner, the Committee led the Society beyond the consideration of government-sponsored, mandatory health coverage into a broader political and ethical agenda. The Committee's 1950 annual report reflects this mission:

> "In the present fight we have not only external enemies but also internal enemies and our very basic liberties are being threatened more dangerously from within than without. In the fight against state medicine, your Committee has found that most of our members are with us in spirit but not in action...The few who have complained and criticized our methods, we feel are really on the other side. That is of course their privilege, but when we do find definitely that people are against us (and some of them talk one way and act another), it is my feeling that no attempt should be made to molly-coddle or appease them, but that they should be dealt with in a direct fashion, recognizing of course, that they have as much right to their opinions as the rest of us."

The Society went on to oppose federal aid to medical schools, a Federal School Bill and a Federal Housing Bill. Dr. Koontz prepared a Resolution that the Society form a committee of seven to "handle members of the Society who have been, or may be, convicted of felonies, high crimes or misdemeanors, such as bring disrepute on the medical community." The committee was established, but there were questions about the latitude which would be given it. Dr. Alfred Blalock, who had served as the Society's first post-war President, expressed the opinion that any blanket rule would be a mistake and that Dr. Koontz's report should be rejected. Dr. Chesney agreed, asking "whether this would mean that action would be taken automatically against any member of the Society..." More discussion ensued, and though Dr. Koontz attempted to qualify the extent of his Committee's power by removing the word "misdemeanor," the resolution was soundly rejected. The proposal was rewritten, giving expelled members the right to reapply for membership one year after their expulsion, but it too was declined.

If the scope of the Committee on Public Education's mission was not clear before, it became so in the 1952 annual report, in which Dr. Koontz voiced his satisfaction that the Committee had been effective in fighting "socialism and socialized medicine." He warned, however, that "The battle is not finished...The menace of government control has been slowed, but not stopped." Dr. Koontz cited the threat posed by the power granted to the Social Security Administration to determine who qualified for assistance, as either partially or fully disabled,. He urged that the United States dissolve its membership in the International Labor Organization.

At the peak of influence of the McCarthy committee in Washington, an application for membership in the Baltimore City Medical Society was made which dramatically brought the national issue to Baltimore. Dr. Ruth Bleier applied for membership in early 1953, and was at first approved by the Board of Censors, the committee which reviewed each application. She had passed every state examination and was in every way a legitimate member of the professional medical community. There were no grievances filed against her, she did not own a drug store nor did she practice osteopathy or chiropractic. That was all that was normally required for membership. It was revealed, however, that in 1951 Dr. Bleier had been called to testify before the Senate Committee on Un-American Activities, in her position as Chairman of the Maryland Committee for Peace. The Board of Directors of Sinai Hospital earlier expressed the opinion that Dr. Bleier ought not be admitted. Her testimony to the Senate Committee was read to those gathered in the Friedenwald Room of the MedChi building on Cathedral Street, and the Board of Censors reversed its decision, denying her membership to the Baltimore City Medical Society.

"The ultimate irony is that my interest in, and work for, peace, an effort to save human life and prevent the barbarism of mass murder, should be used as grounds to deny my membership in a medical society whose highest dedication is the saving of life," Dr. Bleier objected. She vowed to protest the decision to prevent her from joining the Society, but to little effect.

The final chapter in the Committee on Public Medical Education's unofficial role as political ethics monitor came in June, 1956. It had been reported to Dr. Koontz that a recent graduate from medical school, a Dr. Byrne "was going to sell his house in the Walbrook area to Negroes." The Minutes of the meeting record that "Dr. Koontz felt that this was wrong and this boy ought to be brought before the Executive Board." This was done, and Dr. and Mrs. Byrne gave a good account of themselves, stating that certain members of the Fairmount Association, the neighborhood organization, threatened him that if he sold his house to "undesirables" his medical license might be withheld. The Society's Executive Board reassured the young doctor that his real estate activities had no influence on his eligibility to practice medicine. Dr. Lewis Gundry commented that he "might not like the color of his suit but that could not keep him from practicing medicine if he passed the examination."

Advertising and the Commercialization of Medicine

For the balance of the Eisenhower years, the Baltimore City Medical Society was spared major considerations of ethics and ethical infractions. However, one nagging problem, stubbornly remained on the agenda. Since the dawn of medical societies, it was considered unprofessional to publicize one's services in any way at all, even if the "advertisement" was the simple note that Dr. Albert B. Bradley wished to post in a community newspaper, announcing the opening of his Belair Road office. "There was some discussion," the Minutes of September 17, 1958, recorded. "It was the feeling of the group that Dr. Bradley should be advised against inserting such an advertisement."

It had been forty years since the Society first looked into the practice of publicity for medical practitioners, and at that time they extracted an agreement from the local press to cease printing physicians' names in connection with any case. In the interim years, however, two developments posed this question in a different light. In 1914, when the editors of many Baltimore city-wide and local papers sat down with the Society to fashion a policy regarding medical reporting, a small fraction of Baltimore homes had telephones. In addition, in the years just before World War I, general practitioners still made up the majority of practicing physicians. Both of those things reversed their course at the end of the next war.

So in February, 1957, when local ophthalmologists came to the Society seeking a decision on the ethics of listings in phone books, the matter of advertising again sparked discussion. Dr. Herman K. Goldberg wrote that the Society's Eye Section voted affirmatively to grant ophthalmologists the privilege of being listed in the yellow pages along with regular physicians and surgeons, with an additional notation: "Practice Limited to Ophthalmology." Dr. John Classen was instructed to write to the ophthalmologist to advise him that his request would be in violation of Society policies, and to send a similar letter to the telephone company educating the advertising representatives about the policy.

Dr. Goldberg was not content to let the matter die. The following month he appeared in person at a meeting of the Society's Executive Board to plead his case. "Dr. Goldberg stated that the ophthalmologists had a special problem, namely, the competition from optometrists." The problem with optometrists was that they had no training in the treatment of diseases of the eye, and often simply fitted patients with new glasses who required treatment for an underlying ailment.

A heated discussion of whether this was "advertising" or not followed. One member expressed the opinion that because his patients uniformly had to wait as long as four weeks for an appointment with an ophthalmologist, it was better to leave the consultations up to the general practitioner rather than the yellow pages. "The family doctor acts as a buffer between the patients and the ophthalmologists and thus is able to keep them from getting irate," he theorized.

Within a month the Committee for the Proposed Listing of Ophthalmologists in the Telephone Directory, a group made up of Eye Section members, decided to go ahead with the listing anyway. The Society's Executive Board replied, opining that this would be "an opening wedge for other groups to seek same listings...poor public relations." Eventually, in 1971, practitioners were granted permission to list two specialties in the yellow pages.

Even poorer public relations, in the opinion of the Society's governing Board, was the practice of posting a blue cross emblem on the license tags of a physician's automobile. It was suggested that the public resented seeing these symbols on the bumpers of luxury automobiles, especially when the driver "is guilty of a breach in motoring etiquette." There was also the risk of liability when a physician was stopped to render first aid in the event of an automobile accident, to say nothing of the likelihood that drug addicts would break into the doctor's car in search of drugs or valuables. A May, 1957 resolution said " WHEREAS, public relations of the medical profession is at a low ebb and needs to be improved... RESOLVED, that the physicians of Maryland be urged to remove the blue cross or similar identification tags from their automobiles..."

What to do about the public's perceived resentment of physicians? Hire a public relations firm. That was the conclusion of the Executive Board at the same meeting at which the license tag issue was discussed. Dr. Whitmer Firor pointed out that "it had been shown that States with a good public relations outfit had a very small number of malpractice suits." Dr. Classen thought that a good public relations campaign may strengthen the Society, and serve to "bring factions of the Society together." He was instructed to meet with a representative from a local public relations firm to see what they might offer. Five months later, Dr. Classen reported back, having concluded that the public relations firm was "trying to sell" something, and that their approach was incompatible with the Society's mission. The idea was tabled, public relations matters left to the state Faculty, and this was the last notation of the decade regarding the Ethics Committee.

Developments in medical insurance and government participation in the financing of health care brought the Society back to ethical considerations in 1966. Medical organizations on every level were fresh from the unsuccessful battle against Medicare and Medicaid and continuing their objection to corporate medicine, which they defined as a doctor working for a hospital or industry for a salary, as opposed to billing patients privately. The AMA reluctantly accepted the presence of the federal government in hospital accounting, but the state Faculty put its foot down when it came to compensation for its practitioner-members. Were a doctor to sign an agreement to be paid by a hospital or a business, and to allow that entity to sell his services, he was deemed by the Medical and Chirurgical Faculty to be in violation of its Code of Ethics and that doctor could be prosecuted.

The issue was nothing new. In 1959, the Maryland Chapter of the American College of Surgeons declared that "many hospitals are engaging in unethical corporate practice of medicine by hiring, on salaries, physicians who render treatment to private patients, part or all of the fees ... are then being collected and/or kept by the hospital rather than by the individual physician responsible for the treatment." They labeled this "the corporate practice of medicine by hospitals." The excuse given by hospitals, in Baltimore notably City Hospitals, was that the only way to retain physicians "dedicated to teaching" was to offer them an alternative to a time-consuming private practice. In addition, these hospitals continued to admit private patients and collect fees "ostensibly for research," but actually used for hospital general expenses and physicians' salaries. The result, the College of Surgeons proclaimed, was "Municipal Institutions chartered for the care of indigent patients perverting their purpose by permitting the elective admission of private patients and seeking millions of dollars of taxpayers' money to accommodate them..." In 1959, it was estimated that the Baltimore affiliate of Blue Shield had made over $350,000 in such payments, arguably in violation of its charter.

A reorganization of Baltimore City Hospitals in 1962 was to have put an end to this practice, opening the doors of the hospital to all practitioners, reforming the hospital's procedures and hopefully returning it to its rightful place as a hospital for the city's poor. By putting the brakes on the admission of private, elective patients at the city's only municipally-operated charity hospital, these patients would be redirected to the city's private hospitals where physicians were not on the payroll and thus retained their independence.

But it had not worked, and in 1966 the Society was drawn into a dispute with the state medical Faculty which called on the carpet not only hospital administrators and medical schools but its own members for that which it called unethical corporate medical practices. A questionnaire went out to every Faculty member, 3,300 in all, asking in effect that the member turn him or herself in for engaging in such arrangements with hospitals. Some 2,000 physicians responded, many confused and angry about the Faculty's inquiry into their practices and concerned about the potential for ethical breaches.

The Medical and Chirurgical Faculty wished to create an investigative committee that would have the authority to define ethical vs. unethical conduct, investigate cases presented before it, prosecute ethical infractions and prescribe penalties. Dr. Thomas Turner, Dean of the Medical Faculty at Hopkins, at a Society meeting to discuss the Faculty's upcoming special meeting on the subject, reminded members that expulsion from the AMA for ethical violations carried heavy penalties - financial hardship, legal implications and loss of good reputation. The state medical organization sought Society support, but there were reservations.

This was a grave matter, as the questionnaire made clear. Its goal was a Faculty-determined mechanism for suspension or expulsion of members for what it defined as unethical conduct. It also indicated that members could be suspended simply for not returning the questionnaire. At the root of the problem, as it was identified by the Faculty's Professional Fee Fund Committee, was the old contention that corporate medicine was being practiced at Baltimore City Hospitals in spite of the 1962 reorganization. The physicians functioning within the hospital's "closed" structure were being paid directly by the hospital. If that was happening at City Hospital, it was likely to be the practice at other hospitals as well, and it was in the interpretation of the Faculty clearly in violation of AMA principles:

"A physician should not dispose of his services under terms

which...interfere with or impair the free and complete exercise of his medical judgement...or cause a deterioration in the quality of medical care."

Members were concerned that hospitals were considering hiring full time medical staffs, "effectively dispensing with the private surgeon and depriving patients of his [sic.] free choice of physician when hospitalized." It was the classic debate between a patient's paying his doctor directly or the doctor being paid by the hospital. Private physicians believed that the latter restricted the patient's choice of doctor. Johns Hopkins Hospital indeed had full-time physicians on the staff, who did not have separate private practices and whose income was provided exclusively by Hopkins. Johns Hopkins also shared with the University of Maryland the operation of Baltimore City Hospitals. Dr. Turner warned that "any net cast for Hopkins faculty will catch a lot of other fish, too...Imagine the great Dr. William Welch being harassed by a regulation like this."

In the end, the Society voted against approval of the Fee Fund Committee Report and the Faculty By-Laws change that would grant it the overwhelming power demanded. A year later, in its Reports to the House of Delegates, the state Faculty backed off its hard line stance with a new definition:

"Historically, the term 'ethical' has been used...to refer to matters involving (1) Moral principles; (2) Customs and usages of the medical profession; and (3) matters of policy not necessarily involving issues of morality in the practice of medicine.

Unethical conduct involving *moral principles*...calls for disciplinary action such as censure, suspension or expulsion...Failure to conform to the customs and usages...may call for disciplinary action depending upon the circumstances...In matters strictly of a policy nature, a physician who disagrees with the position of the American Medical Association...is entitled to the freedom and protection of his point of view."

Minor issues of ethics arose from time to time, but for the most part the role of setting and enforcing standards of professional conduct moved to the state and national level. In 1969, the Society questioned whether it was proper for a practitioner to bill a patient for laboratory tests not done in the doctor's office. The determination, coming a year later, was that the physician could bill, for example, for drawing blood but not for any tests completed by an outside contractor. A Peer Review Committee was created under the leadership of Dr. Katherine Borkovich in 1970, but most of the complaints handled by that Committee as well as the Professional Relations Committee were matters of fees and billing rather than ethics.

A panel of three professionals, the AMA's director of ethics, a Hopkins professor and a local clergyman, talked about the application of two centuries of ethical rulings to the more contemporary issues of abortion, genetic engineering and physician-assisted suicide in 1975. Nine years later the Society ruled that a doctor could contribute medical services to be used as a raffle item (presumably by a non-profit organization) only when the service was medically indicated. Clearly, medical ethics, while still important, had taken a back seat to more urgent issues as the Baltimore City Medical Society closed its books on its first 100 years.

"The following arrangements tend to exploit the patient for financial gain and, therefore, constitute an unethical division on fees...Physicians who accept compensation from any source (e.g., pharmacist...) for referral of patients..."

-Ethical statements adopted by
the MedChi Council, June, 1984

"When I set up my practice in the 1960's, a local druggist started giving me ice cream sodas, milkshakes, insinuating that there would be more to come if I sent my patients to him. I started going to a different drugstore."

-Dr. Roland E. Smoot
from a February, 2004 interview

"In every back yard...there was a cesspool...and open sewers which ran along the curbs of every street. All other waste water found its way into the gutters, whence eventually it might be let into a storm water drain. Such drains all emptied either into the Jones Falls or directly into the Basin. The Falls thus became a great open sewer - often tinted a sickly blue on Monday - discharging its malodorous contents into the inner harbor whose waters bubbled constantly as they engendered the noxious gases of putrefaction.

Nor was that the worst of the situation. The visitor could not see the water supply system..."

-from *Baltimore on the Chesapeake*
by Hamilton Owens

> *"Those who have suffered most from the Fever dwell on a soil made by their own hands...A foul core in the heart of the City."*
>
> -A report of the Physicians of the Second Dispensary in Baltimore, 1820

Public Health and Sanitation in Baltimore

Though physicians in the eighteenth century knew nothing about bacteriology - the work of Pasteur, Lister and Koch was still a century in the future - many had already made a connection between waste and disease. During the Revolutionary War, Baltimore Doctor Frederick Weisenthal found that wounded soldiers stood a better chance of survival if they didn't have to lie on another man's soiled bedding. Thus, from the very earliest days of professional medical organizations the mission of improved public health was of prime importance. If doctors could not cure yellow fever and bilious fever, they could at least hope to prevent the epidemics that decimated Fells Point and Old Town working populations by advocating for sanitation, clean water and eventually pasteurized milk.

In 1793, the first three local government health officials were appointed in Baltimore, to protect the city from a yellow fever epidemic that was then raging in Philadelphia. Barriers were erected on the road from Philadelphia to prevent the passage of infected travelers. The Baltimore City Health Department is thus the oldest continually operating health department in the world. The City's 1796 charter recognized the importance of public sanitation, empowering the City to pass any ordinance "necessary to preserve the health of the city; prevent and remove nuisances; to prevent the introduction of contagious diseases within the city and within three miles of the same." The first Board of Commissioners of Health was appointed in 1797. Baltimore was the nation's fourth largest city when it was incorporated in 1796. The population stood at 13,524 and was growing dramatically. Along with that growth came increasing problems of public health.

It was an epidemic of yellow fever in 1819 that resulted in the first reorganization of the Board of Health. The Baltimore Medical Society proposed a plan to the Baltimore City Council that was eventually adopted. In the Society's plan was a laundry list of evils that needed correction to prevent the scourge that, in 1819, infected 1200 residents of the city's low-lying areas. Society President Dr.

Ashton Alexander recommended that the docks and wharves be cleaned every spring, that rotting material in the streets either be removed or paved over and that the paving be done in such a fashion as to create drainage on either side of the roadway. Basements were either to be prohibited or in some fashion monitored to make sure that they remained dry throughout the year. Strict quarantine not only upon ships' passengers arriving from distant ports, but also upon the vessels' cargos was recommended.

"The Yellow Fever epidemic will discourage the growth of cities ... & I view cities as pestilential to the morals, the health and the liberties of man."
-Thomas Jefferson, in a letter to Dr. Benjamin Rush
September, 1800

A review of the history of epidemic disease in Baltimore would lead one to ask how it was possible for anyone at all who lived in Fells Point, Old Town, along the banks of the Jones Falls, or within olfactory range of the Basin to live into his or her adult years.

1757 - Smallpox outbreaks in Annapolis were so great that the legislature met in Baltimore. The disease spread to Baltimore, and the Governor declared August 12 a day of "fasting, humiliation and prayer."

1794 - A severe epidemic of yellow fever killed an estimated 360 Baltimoreans, from a population of about 18,000.

1797 - In spite of the city's effort to quarantine itself from Philadelphia, where a summertime "malignant fever" was spreading, yellow fever again swept the streets of east Baltimore. One good thing came from the episode: Dr. John Beale Davidge wrote his landmark book on the disease in 1798.

1800 - Due to "an epidemic constitution of the air," yellow fever again raged, despite physicians' attempts to keep it at bay with purgatives and castor oil.

1802 - The Medical and Chirurgical Faculty passed a resolution endorsing smallpox vaccination. "From the year 1750 until 1800 the disease was rarely absent...(it) frequently ravaged the towns and country with great virulence."

1808, 1819 - More than 2200 deaths from yellow fever were reported in 1819, most of which were traced to the Point. It was noted that visiting Fells Point by night, rather than in the daytime, increased one's chances of contracting the fever dramatically.

1832 - "In the city of Baltimore there died of cholera...eight hundred and fifty three persons, a very great majority of whom were the most worthless; but a few of our best citizens were its victims." (Dr. Horatio G. Jameson, consulting physician to Baltimore City)

1849 - Eighty three cases of typhus were sent to the Almshouse, "invariably from filthy and unwholesome localities."

1902 - Dr. William Osler asked the Mayor "What are we doing for the 10,000 consumptives who are living today in our midst?"

In 1911, the year the sewage system was put into operation, Baltimore's water supply was chlorinated. The rate of typhoid fever plummeted. Rates of death from cholera, scarlet fever and whooping cough also declined, following the introduction of water from the Gunpowder River to the taps of Baltimore City.

Tuberculosis still raged, but in 1910 a Commission proposed a strategy of prevention. But clean water, streets free of rotting debris, increased diligence regarding incoming freight and passengers, coupled with the advances of science and communications failed to stop epidemic disease.

1918 - "Spanish" influenza swept Baltimore and the world. Over 500,000 Americans died. Streetcar tokens were washed in an antiseptic solution before being reused. Mayor James H. Preston was quoted as saying that aiming a cough or a wad of spittle at a person was as serious as aiming a gun.

Presently, although the words "epidemic" and "pandemic" may be flagrantly abused by the media, if one is to take the press literally, Baltimore is still deluged by "epidemics" of homicide, HIV/AIDS (In 2003, second only to homicide in the cause of death of Baltimoreans under the age of 25), congenital syphilis (In 1996 and 1997, Baltimore had the highest rate of any city in the nation), heroin use (stubbornly persisted in Baltimore throughout the 1990's), and Hepatitis C (in 1999, the rate of Hepatitis C infection of chronic drug users in Baltimore was nearly twice the national average).

Dr. Alexander proposed a means of public sanitation unique to the times, calling for the repeal of "laws restricting hogs running at large and the throwing of kitchen offal into the streets...as these animals destroy vast quantities of such materials which if suffered to undergo composition might become pernicious to health." A century later a similar effort was made to employ the limitless appetites and digestive capacities of hogs, when in 1920 the city bought 160 acres 11 miles from town and established a piggery. Fifteen thousand pigs were installed and they happily began converting 25 pounds of garbage daily to one pound of pork. The taxpayers and city fathers were ecstatic with the plan until the piggery's manager reached the first slaughter season, killed his porcine workers, sold the meat and absconded with $15,000.

The Baltimore Medical Association and its peer organizations were less involved in sanitation issues, and more focused on treatment of people, both in hospitals and in day-to-day practice. Perhaps because the greatest medical legacy of the Civil War was the physical reorganization of hospitals and a rethinking of hospital management, the societies which were founded in the years just after the war tended to concentrate on the development of hospital facilities. In 1872 the Association issued a resolution calling for a special hospital for contagious and infectious diseases to serve both indigents and paying patients, albeit in separate wards.

On June 26, 1876 Dr Scott read "a very interesting and entertaining paper on 'The Basin - Is there a relation between offensive odors and disease?' " Later that year the recurrent battle with yellow fever was a topic, and the Association blamed the outbreak in September,

1876 on sanitary conditions in the city. Dr. Abraham Arnold, the Association's President in 1871, related the story of a pocket of yellow fever in east Baltimore: "The disease has existed for about 6 weeks and about 80% of the number have died...The infected region was in a miserable sanitary condition." The speaker theorized that yellow fever was brought by a cook on board a barque that had been detained at quarantine. Dr. John F. Monmonier asked if the deceased had, as he recalled from the 1854 epidemic, "spleens like blackberry jam." No action was taken, no call to the City to clean up the infected neighborhoods.

For the most part, it was the state Medical and Chirurgical Faculty that took the lead in public health initiatives in the last quarter of the nineteenth century. The Faculty's Committee on Sanitation had worked with the City to establish a bacteriological laboratory in 1896 and lobbied for local laws regulating the purity of milk, improvement of conditions in sweatshops and school-wide vaccination. The Committee was instrumental in the establishment of the Walters Public Baths, made possible by the generosity of philanthropist Henry Walters. The first bath opened in Baltimore in May, 1900, at the corner of Central Avenue and East Baltimore Street. The publication of *The Medical Annals of Maryland* in 1903, the most exhaustive study of the history of organized medicine in Maryland to that date, acknowledged the new focus on public health: "As prevention is better, more easily secured and more certain than cure, our efforts are increasingly directed to that, and in no respect does modern medicine contrast so strongly with that of former times as in the marvelous progress made in this field."

Nationally, states and cities were becoming more involved in the financial affairs of their citizens, and the success of local economies in large part hinged on the cities' public services. Demands for service from local government resulted in a new Baltimore City Charter in 1898. The document ended the monopoly held by ward-level pols on constituent services, centralizing most day-to-day functions at City Hall. The decision making shifted from those with little professional expertise but plenty of street level political clout to engineers, trained inspectors and planners.

Sanitary conditions reflected the most obvious failure of Baltimore's Public Works Department. But despite repeated initiatives to do something about the sewage that sluggishly flowed down each side of every Baltimore street and alley and floated out to the Chesapeake on the outgoing tide, it was the Baltimore Fire of 1904 which eventually forced City officials to take action. Special commissions on public sanitation and drinking water quality had been convened in 1859, 1881 and 1897, but their work was for naught. Even when

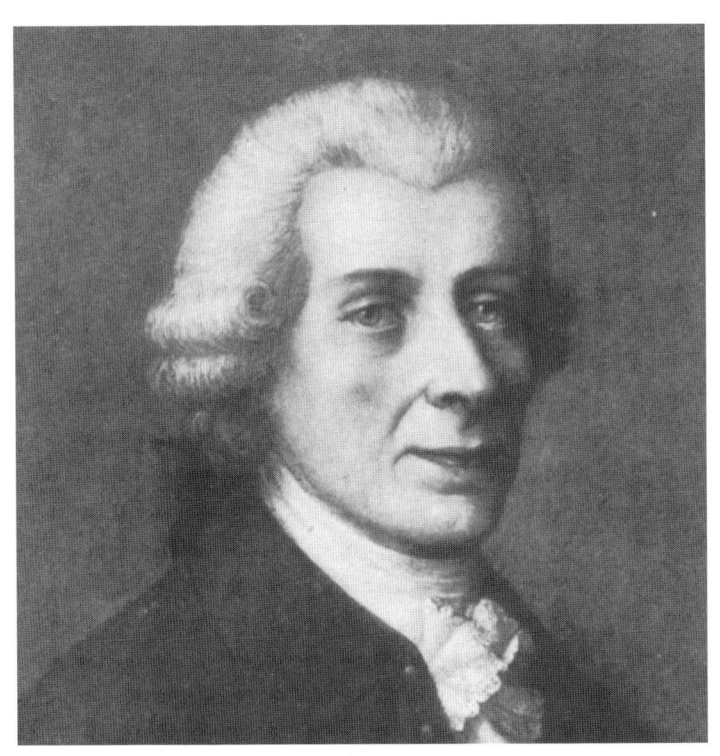

Dr. Charles Wiesenthal, called the father of medical education in Baltimore and President of the first local medical society. From a portrait painted by his son, Andrew Wiesenthal, M.D.

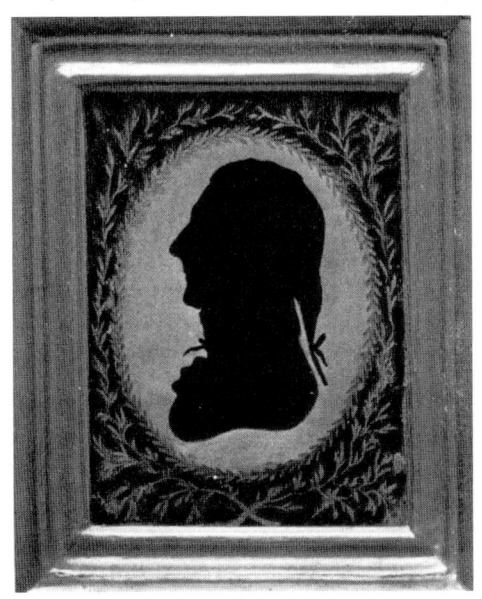

Dr. George Buchanan was one of the founders of the first Baltimore medical society as well as a founder of the Medical and Chirurgical Faculty of Maryland.

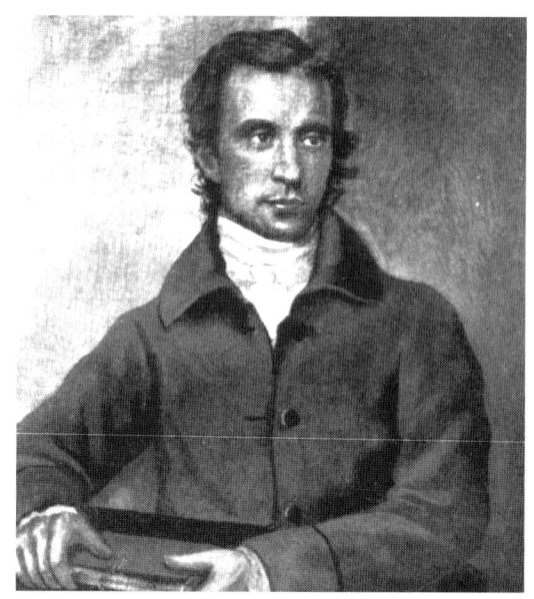

Dr. Samuel Baker is credited with being the father of the library of the Medical and Chirurgical Faculty of Maryland. In addition, he was the first President of the Medico-Chirurgical Faculty (not the state organization) in 1832.

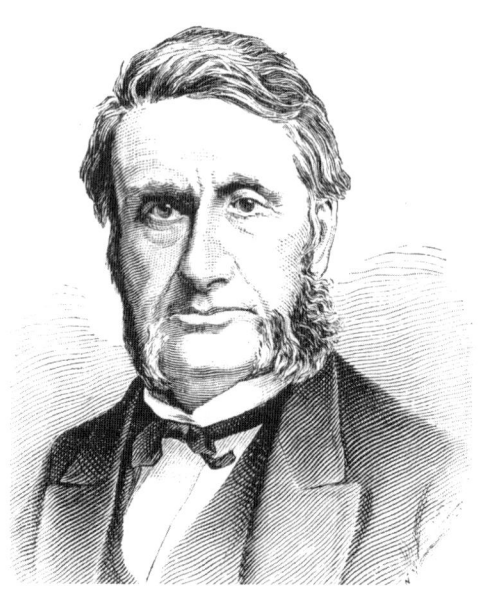

John L. Yeates, M.D. presided over the Medical and Surgical Society of Baltimore from 1855-1856.

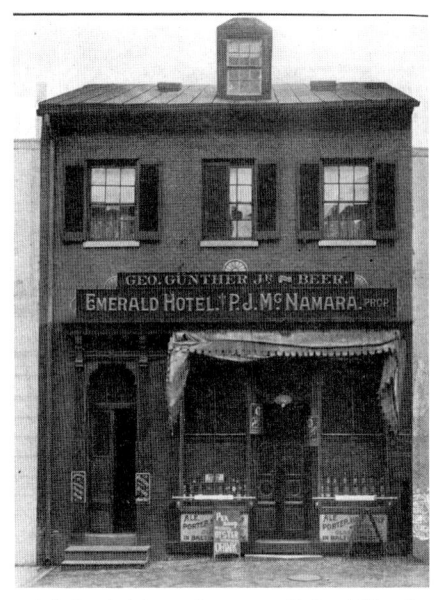

A federal style rowhouse on Calvert Street was the first home of the Baltimore Medical Association. The Association shared space with the state Faculty. The hotel was not there in 1866.

CONSTITUTION

AND

BY-LAWS

OF THE

BALTIMORE

Medical Association

OF

BALTIMORE.

BALTIMORE:
PRINTED BY FREDERICK A. HANZSCHE,
234 BALTIMORE STREET.

1866.

The 1866 Constitution of the Baltimore Medical Association, published in a slim volume scarcely larger than a postcard.

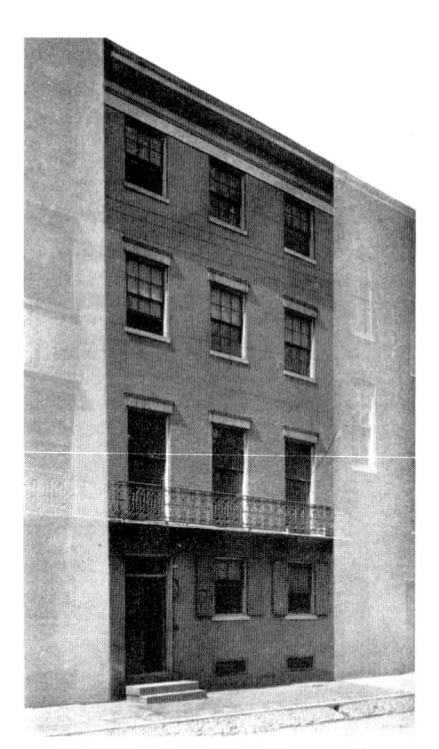

No. 60 Courtland Street became the home of the Baltimore Medical Association in 1869. Since razed, the site is now occupied by Mercy Hospital.

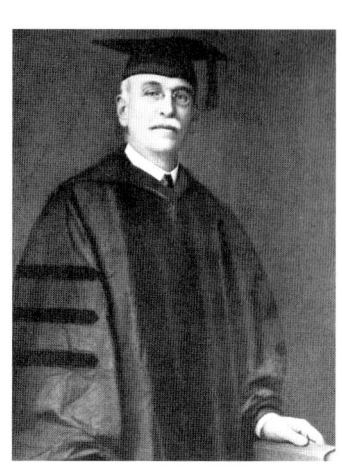

Eugene Fauntleroy Cordell, M.D., author of a centennial history of the University of Maryland School of Medicine

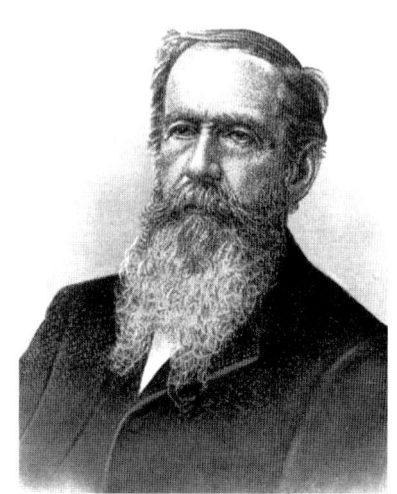

John R. Quinan. M.D., an early Baltimore medical historian, wrote *The Medical Annals of Maryland* in 1874.

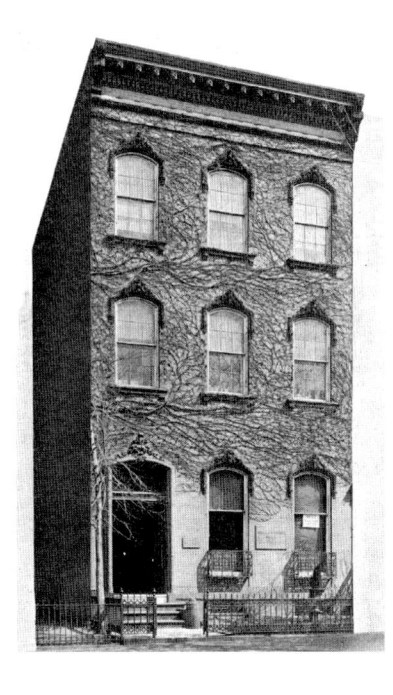

In 1896, the Baltimore Medical Association moved to the new headquarters of the Medical and Chirurgical Faculty of Maryland, in this North Eutaw Street rowhouse.

BALTIMORE, April 12, 1904.

DEAR DOCTOR:

The arrangements for reorganizing the MEDICAL AND CHIRURGICAL FACULTY OF MARYLAND in accordance with the new plans of the AMERICAN MEDICAL ASSOCIATION have been about completed. It is necessary now that the members residing in Baltimore City shall meet to form an organized local branch of the State society, and you are earnestly requested to attend such a meeting at the Hall, 847 N. Eutaw St., Friday, April 15, at 8.30 P. M.

H. O. REIK, M. D.
Chairman Com. on Revision of Constitution.

Following the reorganization of the state medical Faculty, this postcard was mailed to every physician in Baltimore to announce the creation of a new Baltimore City society. The Medical and Surgical Association of Baltimore, the result of the merger of two other groups, was active in 1904, meeting at the Faculty headquarters.

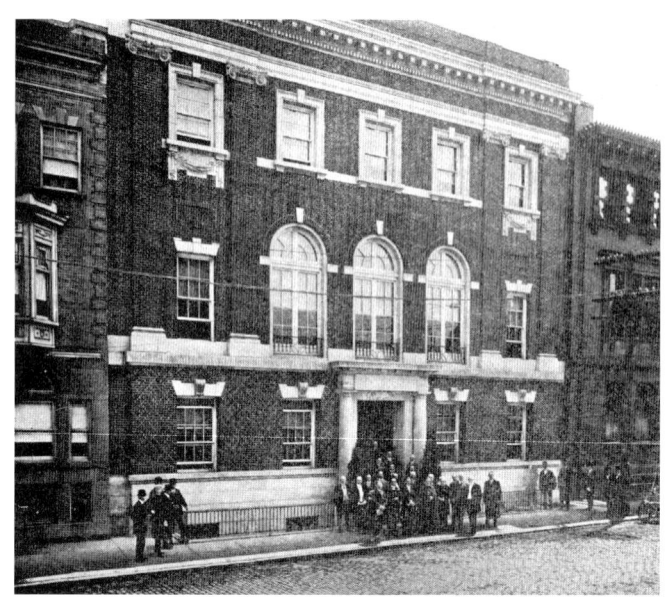

Members of the Medical and Chirurgical Faculty gather in front of their new building for its 1908 dedication. The BCMS met here from 1908 until 1974, moving back in 2001.

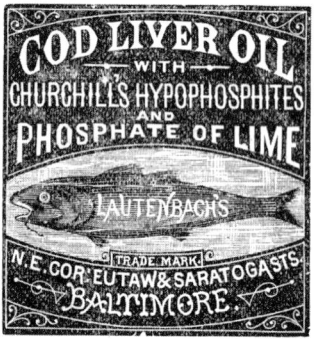

LAUTENBACH'S

ROBT. LAUTENBACH, Pharmacist.

Dear Sir:—I have used your preparation of Cod Liver Oil with Churchill's Hypophosphites and Phosphate of Lime with satisfaction and success in cases of Consumption, Bronchitis, and Catarrh.

Very respectfully,
WILBUR P. MORGAN, M. D.,
175 Saratoga St.

Balt more, October 1st, 1875.

Dear Sir:—I cheerfully recommend R. Lautenbach's preparation of Cod Liver Oil with Churchill's Hypophosphites and Phosphate of Lime; having used it with marked good effect. N. G. RIDGELY, M. D., 352 Madison Avenue.

Experience in the use of R. Lautenbach's Cod Liver Oil with Churchill's Hypophosphites and Phosphate of Lime, has induced me to consider it to be the most pleasant and effective of that class of important remedies. W. G RIDER, M. D., 87 Mulberry Street.

With permission I refer to the following for further testimony:

Prof. A. P. SMITH, 45 Franklin Street.
JUDSON GILMAN, 172 Saratoga Street.
E. M. REID, 245 N. Fremont Street.
J. H. HOUCK, 75 E. Baltimore Street.
Prof S. C. CHEW, 141 Lanvale Street,
E. F MILHOLLAND, 279 W. Lombard St
and numerous others.

WHOLESALE BY

BALTIMORE.
THOMSEN & MUTH,
W. H. BROWN & BRO.
A. VOGELER, SON & CO.

WASHINGTON, D. C.
STOTT & CROMWELL,

NEW YORK.
W. H. SHIEFFELIN & CO.
McKESSON & ROBBINS.
PHILADELPHIA.
JOHNSON HOLLOWAY & COWDEN.

Orders for the above Preparations, Drugs, Medicines, etc., through the mail or otherwise, will receive prompt attention.

Lautenbach's Pharmaceutical Laboratory.
Established, 1857.

1-u

Long before the BCMS stood up to the patent medicine industry, this ad appeared in a July, 1877 issue of the Maryland Medical Journal.

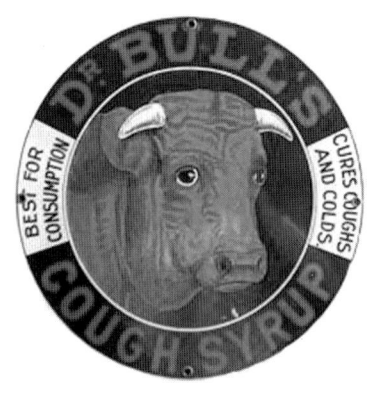

When the Baltimore City Medical Society took on the patent medicine industry in 1908, the A.C. Meyer Company of Baltimore, maker of *Dr. Bull's Cough Syrup* stood in opposition to new regulations that would have required makers to list the ingredients of their products on their labels.

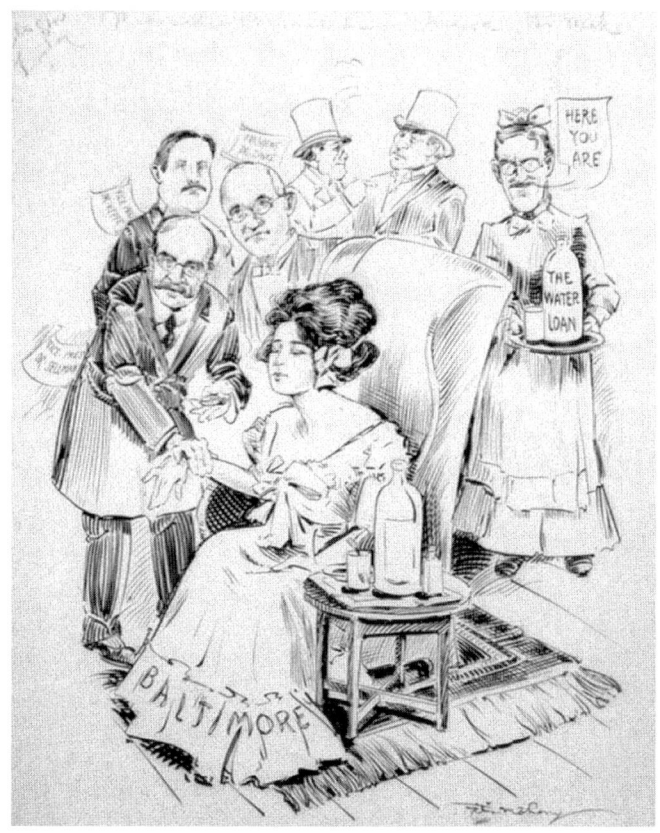

The American Association of Obstetricians and Gynecologists held its annual meeting in Baltimore in September, 1908, and joined with the Baltimore City Medical Society in supporting the Water Loan to provide city residents with pure drinking water. This political cartoon, "Medical Convention in Town This Week - the Doctors Agree she Needs Pure Water," appeared in the September 24, 1908 issue of the *American Star*. Mayor J. Barry Mahool is wearing the apron, delivering pure water to Baltimore.

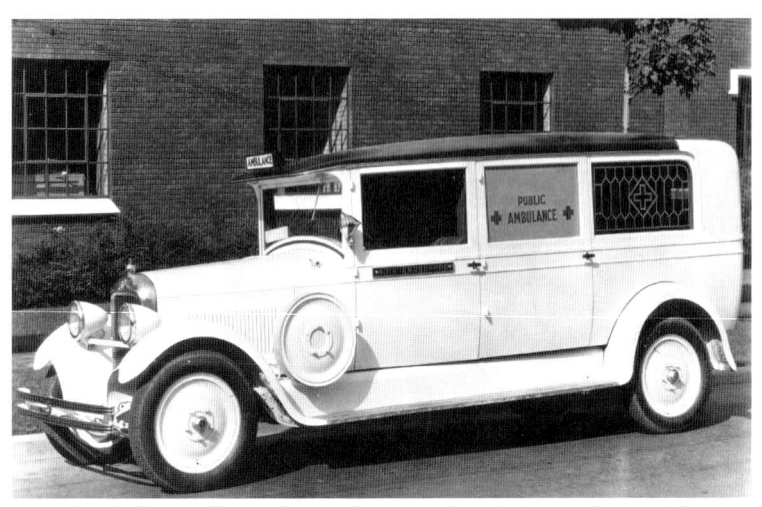

The Baltimore City Medical Society urged the city to establish a public ambulance service in 1927. Three Studebaker ambulances, like the 1927 model above, plus 3 Buick ambulances made up the first fleet. The service was operated by the Baltimore City Fire Department.

Baltimore City Medical Society
1211 Cathedral Street
Baltimore, Md.

IMPORTANT

A SPECIAL MEETING of the Baltimore City Medical Society (all Sections included) will take place FRIDAY, APRIL 13, 1934 at 8.30 P. M.

The brief report of the Society's Committee on GROUP HOSPITALIZATION INSURANCE will be submitted for consideration; after which, a vote for its acceptance or rejection will be taken.

Warfield T. Longcope, M. D.,   Lawrence R. Wharton, M. D.,
President.   *Secretary.*

When important issues were on the Baltimore City Medical Society agenda, postcards like this were mailed to every member. This 1934 meeting was called to discuss one of the earliest attempts to create government-sponsored hospitalization insurance, a concept against which the Society advocated at every level of government.

THE SAD CASE OF WAITING-ROOM WILLIE

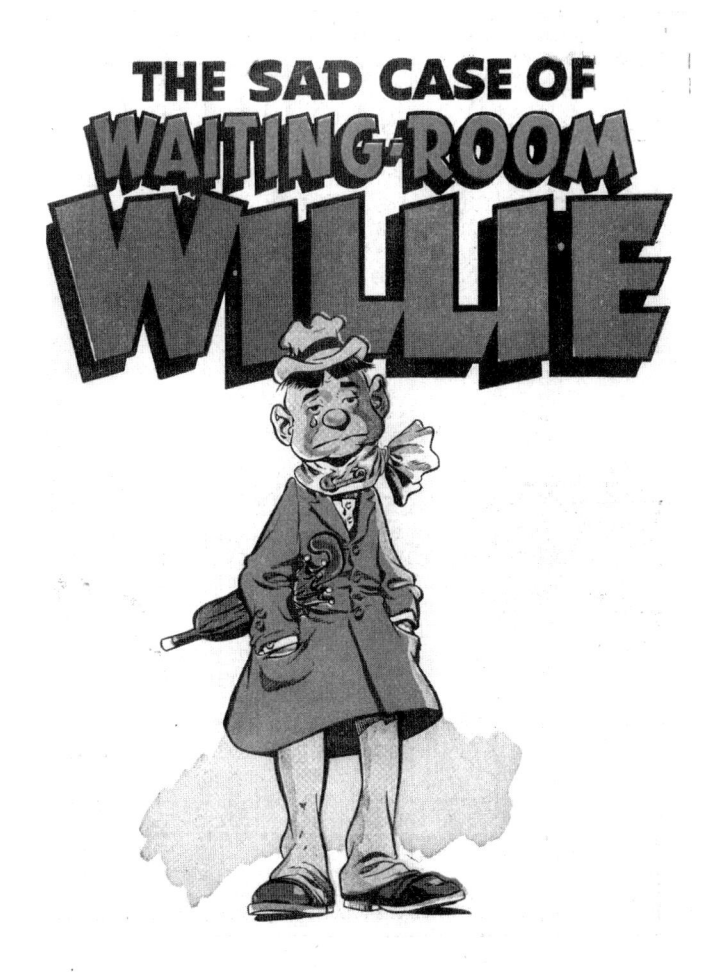

In an effort to educate the public about the threat of socialized medicine, the Baltimore City Medical Society published *The Sad Case of Waiting Room Willie* in 1952. In spite of the comic's simplistic approach, Willie exemplified the position of organized medicine and foretold issues that complicate health care delivery in the 21st century.

BALTIMORE CITY MEDICAL SOCIETY

joint meeting with

MONUMENTAL CITY MEDICAL SOCIETY

1211 Cathedral Street   Baltimore, Maryland

FRIDAY, NOVEMBER 1, 1968, 8:30 P.M.

Problems of Inner City Medicine — 1968

Introductory remarks

Simon H. Carter, Jr., M.D.	D. Frank Kaltreider, M.D.
President	President
Monumental City Medical Society	Baltimore City Medical Society

Private Practice of Medicine   *Hospital Practice of Medicine*

H. Garland Chissell, M.D.   **Torrey C. Brown, M.D.**
General Practitioner   Assistant Professor of Medicine
Baltimore   Johns Hopkins University School of Medicine

BUSINESS MEETING

Acceptable for 1 hour Category I Credit by the American Academy of General Practice

---

BCMS made overtures to the Monumental City Medical Society as early as 1940, inviting members to scientific sessions. This announces a 1968 joint meeting of the two societies.

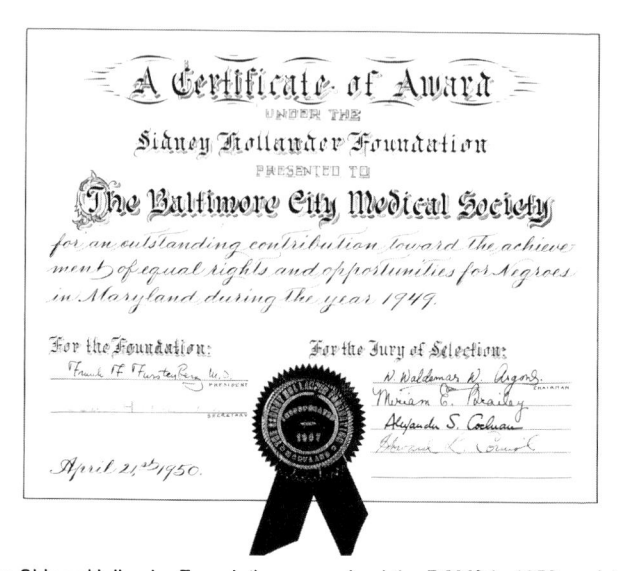

A Certificate of Award
UNDER THE
Sidney Hollander Foundation
PRESENTED TO
The Baltimore City Medical Society
for an outstanding contribution toward the achievement of equal rights and opportunities for Negroes in Maryland during the year 1949.

For the Foundation: For the Jury of Selection:

April 21st, 1950.

The Sidney Hollander Foundation recognized the BCMS in 1950, praising the Society's 1949 initiative to grant full membership to African American practitioners.

The Woman's Auxiliary
to the
Baltimore City Medical Society

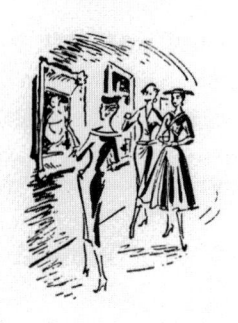

Indoor "SIDEWALK" Art and Christmas Decorations Show and Party

The Women's Auxiliary to the Baltimore City Medical Society was created to plan social events and raise funds for Society programs. Its 1954 holiday sidewalk sale was the first of what became a regular event. The Auxiliary sponsored the Society's first medical school scholarships.

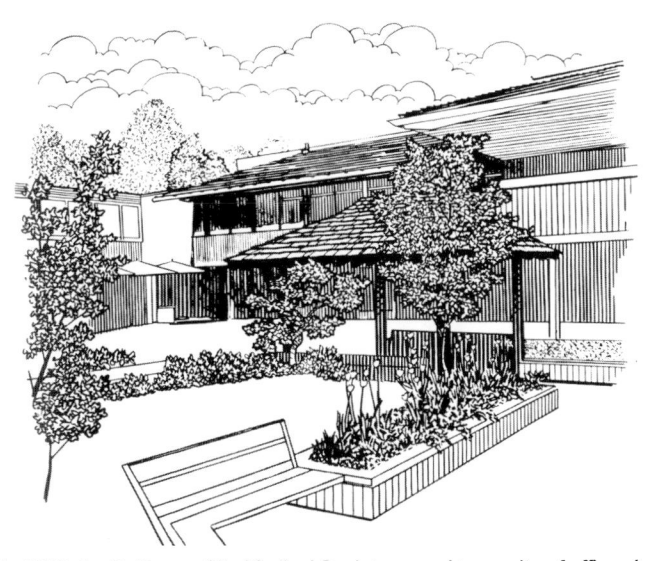

In 1974, the Baltimore City Medical Society moved to a suite of offices in Cross Keys which was its home until 1981. The office's tendency to flood after every major rainstorm made tenancy there difficult. This drawing is from the Society's 1980 *Physicians' Pictorial Register*.

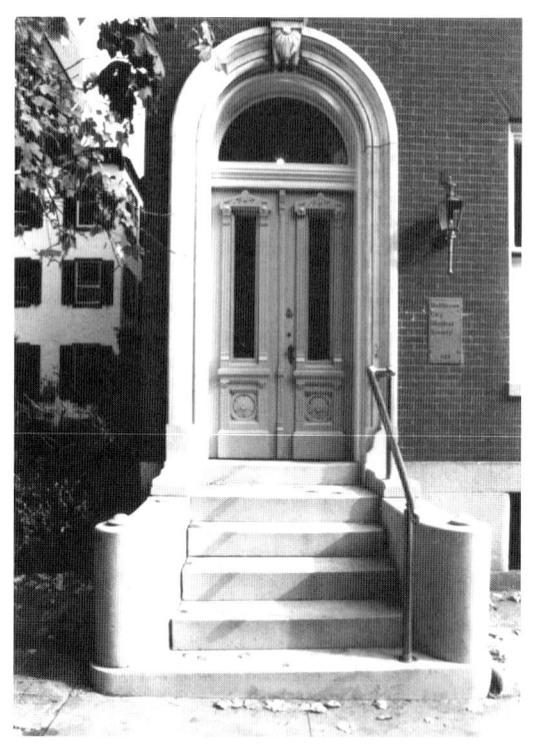

The stately doorway to the Society's Park Avenue office was, typical of Baltimore, framed in white marble. The Italianate style rowhouse was purchased by the Society in 1981.

The Society was an active participant in the Baltimore City Fair. A State Police officer administers a breathalyzer test to a fairgoer at the 1979 City Fair.

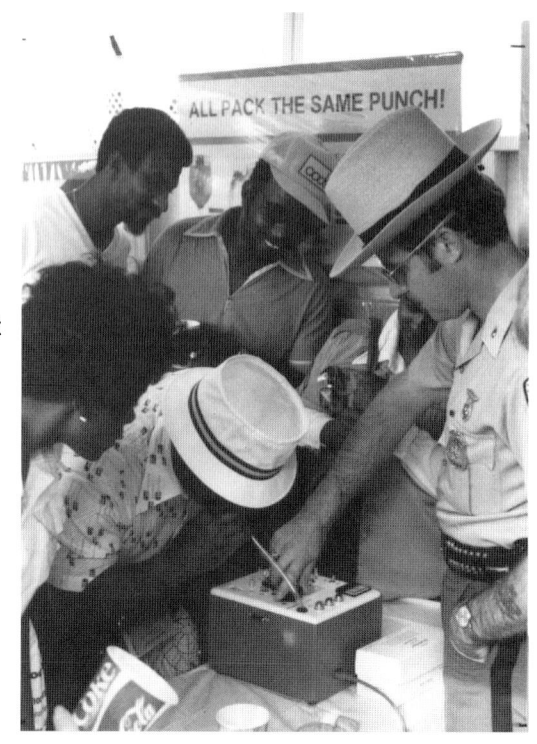

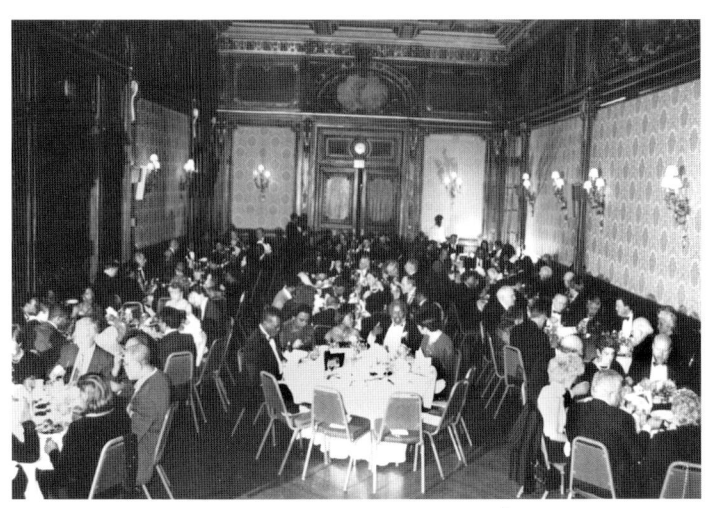

The 2001 investiture of Dr. Reed Winston as the 98th President of the Baltimore City Medical Society was held at the spectacular Engineers Club on Baltimore's Mount Vernon Place. The BCMS office, on Park Avenue, was virtually right around the corner.

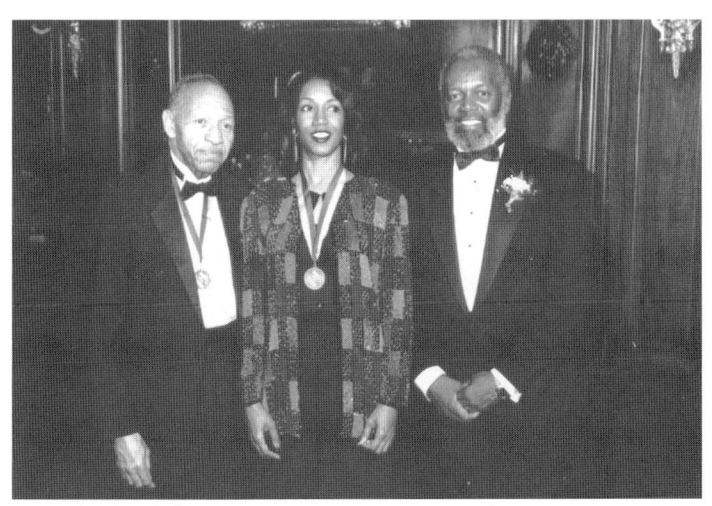

Dr. Roland Smoot (far left) and Dr. Willarda Edwards (center) wear Baltimore City Medical Society Past Presidents' medallions at Dr. Winston's investiture. Dr. Smoot was the first African-American President of both the BCMS and MedChi. Dr. Edwards was the first female African American President of the BCMS.

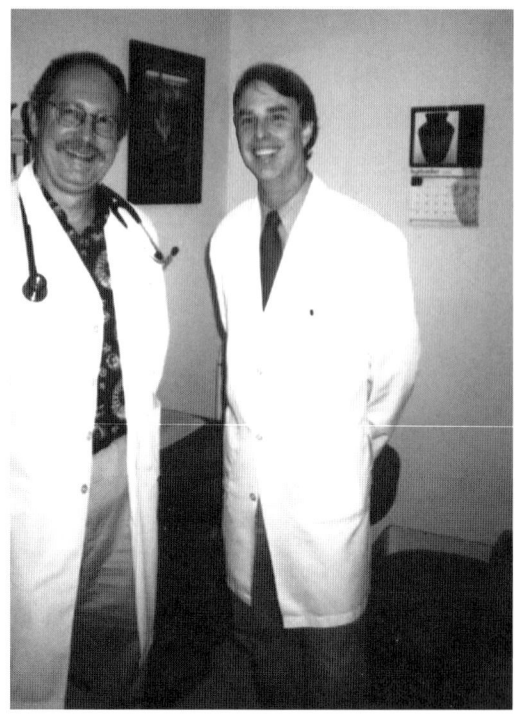

Mini-internships are among the Society's most successful long-term programs. Mr. Jan Houbolt, of the Greater Baltimore Committee (right), spent a day with Dr. Jos Zebley in 2002.

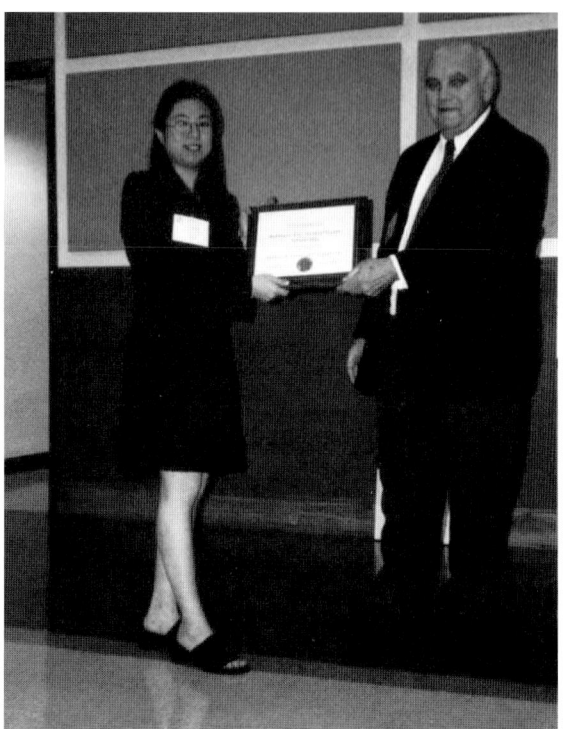

Medical student Cindy KaYee Lee is awarded a check from Dr. Paul Burgan, of the Baltimore City Medical Society Foundation. The scholarship was granted in 2002.

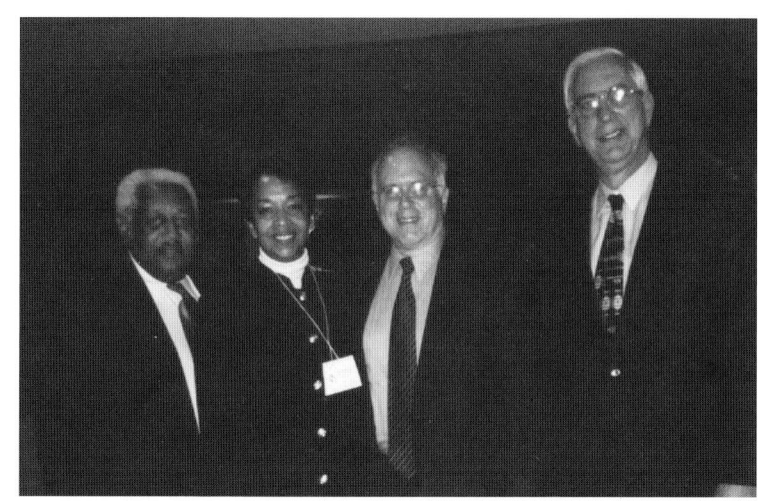

"The Future of Medical Education" was the topic of the BCMS Continuing Medical Education program in February, 2003. Donald Wilson, M.D., Dean of the University of Maryland School of Medicine (far left) and Edward Miller, M.D., Dean of the Johns Hopkins University School of Medicine (far right) addressed the Society. Dr. Eve Higginbotham (second from left) was the current BCMS President. Dr. Murray Kalish (second from right) was the Society's President in 1996.

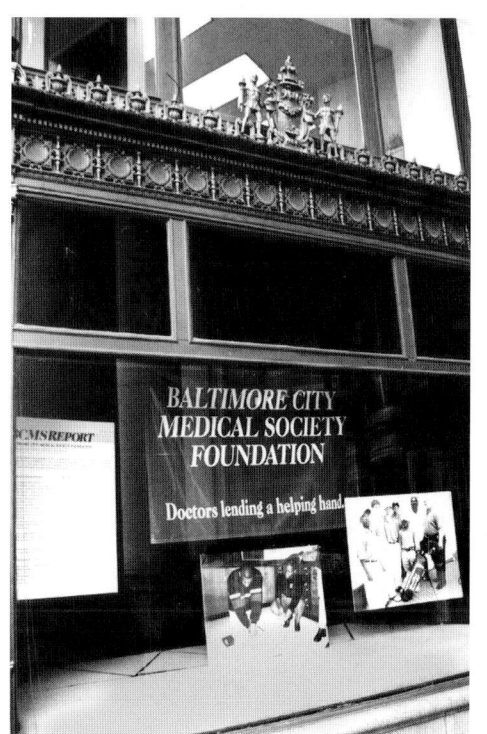

The BCMS Foundation used a window in the Baltimore Gas and Electric Company Building on Liberty Street to inform passersby of its medical education programs.

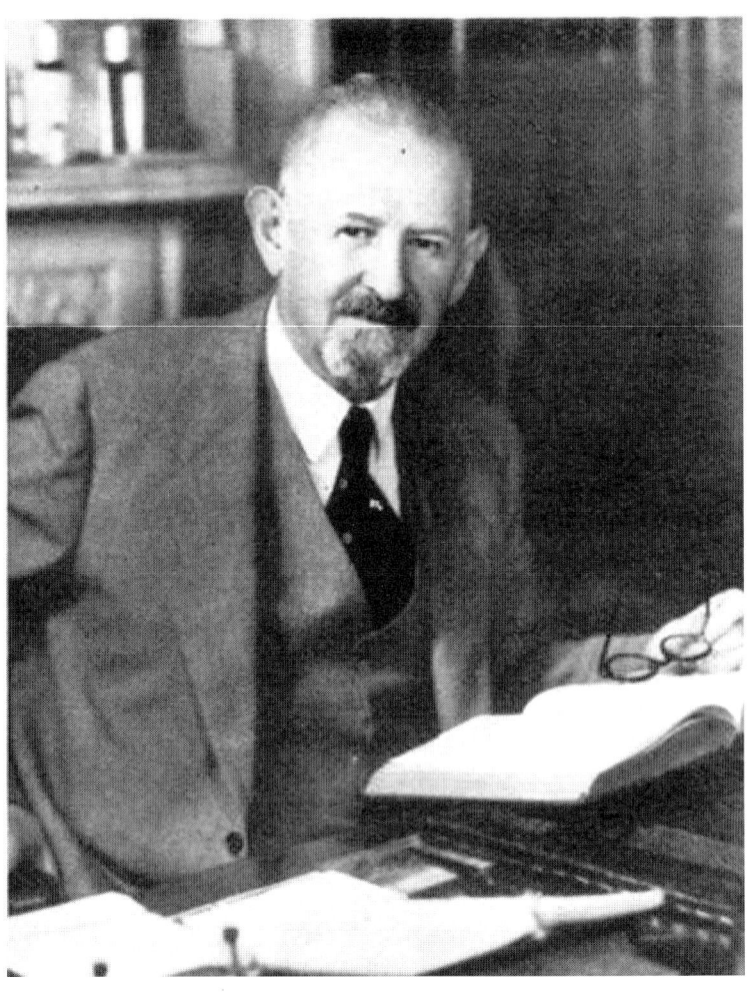

Dr. Harry Friedenwald was the modern Baltimore City Medical Society's first president, and he served a second term beginning in 1913. A specialist in the diseases of the eye and ear, Dr. Friedenwald was also a scholar of Middle Eastern medical history.

the first bond issue to build a modern sewage treatment system was passed, in 1905, the principal motivation was not a particular concern for public health, but for property values. Reconstruction and improvement on plots destroyed in the Great Fire caused the value of those properties to double, and other land valuations in the city followed the path upward. It was estimated in 1904 that cesspools took up 50 acres of land. Between 1900 and 1905 the City issued over 288,000 permits for cesspool pumping, which kept the city's operators of the "Odorless Excavation Apparatus" busy. As long as the City relied on a cesspool system the land over those pools and privies was useless for development.

Public health aside, the city's lack of modern water and waste treatment systems hampered its commercial growth. In the last three decades of the 19th century, Baltimore experienced a three-fold increase in the number of manufacturing concerns and factory workers as the city underwent a metamorphosis from a mercantile to a factory economy. The demand for capital was overwhelming, and Baltimore was in an unfavorable position to attract it, in part because of the lack of municipal services.

The 1905 bond issue authorized $10 million to build the city's first sewage treatment facility. From their pulpits, clergymen instructed their parishioners to support the bond, landlords threatened their tenants with eviction if they did not vote Yes. Public meetings were held, and newspapers enjoined the public to support the measure with headlines like "What It Means to Women." The referendum passed by a huge majority and Mayor E. Clay Timanus appointed a commission to begin design and implementation. It took 11 years to complete, and in that time journalists from all over the world inspected the network of new wastewater and stormwater pipes snaking its way beneath the city. *Leslie's Illustrated Weekly*, a New York publication, included a photograph of five Baltimore dignitaries in a touring car in an article entitled "In the Sewers of Baltimore." The car was in a sewage pipe beneath the corner of Chase and Durham Streets, its passengers posing proudly in straw hats and stiff white collars.

A New Society, A New Committee on Public Health

As the city was determining its course of action, the state's Medical and Chirurgical Faculty was completing a major reorganization. When the Baltimore City reorganization committee met on April 15, 1904, had it been a breezy, warm, spring day, the bitter smell of smoke would have wafted through its open windows on Park Avenue. It would have competed with the aroma of open drains and overflowing cesspools. The Great Fire had scorched Baltimore's financial district just two months earlier, heightening, perhaps, the group's awareness of public health concerns.

One of the Baltimore City Medical Society committees established that day was the Committee on Public Health and Legislation, charged with the "duty to enforce and support the sanitary and medical laws of the State in this City..." Its first action was to join with other citizens and fraternal organizations to protest the dense cloud of black smoke that perpetually hung over the city. Except for a short discussion of the work of City milk dispensaries, that was the first and last public health initiative floated by the Society in two years.

By the Annual Meeting in 1908, the Constitution and By-Laws having been amended as the group gelled and membership reached 514, the Society began to discuss other pertinent matters, including public health. Among the many diseases that periodically swept through Baltimore, typhoid fever remained stubbornly resistant to any search for a cure or even a preventative. That year, Dr. William Welch voiced his discouragement at progress against the disease. It was suspected that typhoid was transmitted through drinking water, but Dr. Welch pointed out that the Potomac River was free from pollution and yet the nation's capital experienced typhoid outbreaks with great regularity. Welch was not convinced that drinking water was the culprit. "We should go slowly in our condemnation of the drinking water in Baltimore," he said.

There was no general agreement, and some in the meeting were resistant to giving the city's water supply a clean bill of health regarding typhoid fever. Some feared that "the pendulum should not swing so far to the other side that water as a carrier be forgotten and other sources be given too much attention." Studies in the District of Columbia, comparing the routes of milkmen who pasteurized their product and sterilized their bottles with the routes of those who did not showed a remarkable difference in the rates of infection. The suggestion was that the milk supply was to blame and that pasteurization and sterilization was the solution.

Henry L. Mencken had already begun publishing the infection rates of the National Typhoid League in *The Sun*. Baltimore always was at the top of the Western Hemisphere list, above even Panama in its rate of infection. Mencken, in his usual acerbic style, blamed City Hall. "A million dollars for a new bridge to the Brooklyn poolroom, but not one cent for typhoid!" In 1911, as the City was preparing to start up the new sewage processing plant on the Bush River, Mencken again coupled death and disease to politics, and City Hall's legendary reluctance to spend money for health:

"Laugh, suckers, laugh!
Down goes the tax rate!
Oh, say, can you see -!
Up goes the death rate!
-by the dawn's early light!"

Water was the subject of the very next Society meeting. Dr. James Bosley, the Commissioner of Health, spoke on the importance of the medical community's support of the upcoming Water Loan. In a meeting a year earlier, Dr. W.W. Ford reported that he had tested tap water in Baltimore City and found it to be polluted. Commissioner Bosley used examples from his own practice to illustrate the effectiveness of clean drinking water in reducing the threat of typhoid fever. Mayor J. Barry Mahool, a legendary Baltimore political figure, described the plans to buy a huge tract in Baltimore County around the present Loch Raven reservoir and seed hundreds of acres as a vegetated buffer around the watershed to absorb agricultural run-off. The original dam, built in 1881, was not adequate to hold the volume of water required by a growing city.

A resolution was agreed upon:

> "WHEREAS, An abundant supply of pure water is of the greatest importance in establishing and protecting the Public Health, and...
>
> WHEREAS, an enabling act, passed in the last Legislature is to be presented to the people...
>
> RESOLVED that the Baltimore City Medical Society hereby endorses the proposed Water Loan..."

Members were exhorted to "use every legitimate means to explain to the citizens the real urgency of the situation and the necessity of going to the polls and voting for the loans." The Water Loan was agreed upon by the voters. Construction of the new Loch Raven Dam began in 1915 and was completed in 1922.

Not content to address only drinking water problems, the Baltimore City Medical Society looked at Baltimore's other drinking problem. Dr. Linthicum admitted that he knew nothing about the subject that he was supposed to discuss in February, 1911: "What is Baltimore Doing For Her Alcoholics?" The topic generated excitement anyway. "A considerable amount of enthusiasm was excited in connection with this subject, so much so that a motion was made that a committee of five be appointed to investigate the subject of alcoholism and see what the Baltimore City Medical Society can do in connection with it." At the next meeting it was determined that whatever the City was doing, it was inadequate, and a Resolution was cast recommending to City Hall that an appropriate hospital for alcoholics be built. Nothing happened, and until 1935 the courts continued to send chronic alcoholics to Baltimore City Hospitals. It was not until 1967, under the leadership of Dr. Roland E. Smoot, the first African American president of both the Society and the state Faculty, that the first alcoholic detoxification unit in a community hospital in the nation was established, at Provident Hospital.

Subsequent sessions found the Society considering a wide range of public health problems, including the implementation of a Hospital Zone Law to attack the problem of noise pollution. The noise Bill became law in 1912. A Special Agent from the United States Department of Justice, with the assistance of a local Volunteers of America captain, gave a presentation in 1913 on "The Relation of the Medical Profession to the Present Vice Crusade," but the Minutes give no indication of which among Baltimore's numerous vices was the topic. A steady schedule of technical topics was occasionally interrupted by public health problems, including calling for the prohibition of "Baby Traffic" in 1916 (through which unwanted babies were sold outside legal adoption and foster care), following a visit to the Society by members of the City's Vice Commission. Later that year Baltimore Commissioner of Health Dr. J.D. Blake brought the matter of an epidemic of poliomyelitis to the Society's attention. Members were urged to attend a public hearing on a proposed Baltimore Milk Ordinance the following year. As the 1918-1919 influenza epidemic was raging, a special meeting was called and representatives from the Health Commission spoke about ways to control communicable diseases.

WHEREAS, the maternal death rate...in Baltimore City is generally recognized as high and has shown comparatively slight changes over a period of years..."
-from a Resolution of the Baltimore City Medical Society
February 15, 1935

When the City of Baltimore announced that it was ending its home obstetrical service and establishing instead a Division of Maternal Hygiene, the Baltimore City Medical Society appointed a Maternal Mortality Survey Committee to study the causes of maternal death in the city. Dr. Huntington Williams, committee chairman and Baltimore City Health Commissioner, forecast in December, 1935 that the study would be carried on "over several years, at the end of which time a final report may be presented to the Medical Society with recommendations dealing with...reducing maternal morbidity rates...in this city."

THE BALTIMORE CITY MEDICAL SOCIETY - A History

The Baltimore Society's landmark study was among the first of its kind in the professional community. The program that set the standard was begun only three years earlier by the Philadelphia County Medical Society, and lasted only until 1934. It distinguished between preventable and non-preventable deaths and explored options to reduce the rate. Baltimore's study followed that model.

Twenty-two years later (more than "several"), the Society committee made its final report. Dr. Williams was still Chair in 1957, and he recommended that the study continue on a statewide basis. Between the institution of the study and 1944 there are but sketchy notes in the Annual Meeting Minutes, with no data. Beginning in 1944, however, regular reports offer a glimpse of the risks of bearing a child in Baltimore:

1944 - Rate of 2.1 deaths per 1,000 live births, an increase over the rate of 1.5 in 1943. (The increase was attributed to a rise in the rate among white mothers, with the rate among African Americans declining).
1945 - Rate declined to 1.7. Only 60% of African American mothers delivered in a hospital setting, as opposed to 89% of white mothers. African American mothers were attended by midwives 9% of the time.
1948 - Rate continued to decline to 1.1. Almost two-thirds were deemed to have been preventable.
1951 - A further drop to .5 was reported, correlating to an increase in hospital births to 93% overall (data no longer broken down by race).
1954 - The rate rose slightly to .75, and details of the causes were outlined. Most were due to hemorrhage and shock. White births still outnumber African American births in Baltimore by nearly 2:1.
1957 - The Society's final report. The rate of mortality for the year stood at .48, a total of 13 deaths. This represents a decline in the rate by 75% since 1944. In 1936, when the data were first collected, there were 52 deaths in the first 9 months alone.

The national rate in 1945 was 1.07 deaths per thousand live births, and by 1960 it had dropped to .37 and has remained almost unchanged since. Baltimore, like all old east coast cities, lagged behind, although it posted a better rate in the reduction of maternal death. Dr. Marsden Wagner, in a 1994 report prepared while he was Director of Women's and Children's Health for the World Health Organization, said that "The reason the maternal mortality fell in the U.S. this century was because of the advent of antibiotics and blood transfusion more than anything else. There is simply no scientific evidence to prove the falling mortality was because birth was moved into the hospital." Dr. Wagner theorized that the rate has remained stubbornly high - the U.S. was 16th in the world in maternal mortality in 2000 - because of increasingly limited access to health care for the working poor. The complexity of finding pre-natal service in America's convoluted system, according to Dr. Wagner, resulted in delays that could change outcomes. The rate among African Americans was 4 times higher than that among whites, matching the degree to which African Americans are uninsured.

World War I monopolized many of the Society's bi-weekly meetings, but after the Armistice was signed a symposium on "Health Conditions in the Schools of Baltimore" was mounted. In the years between the wars, local public health slipped to a lower priority. There were more presentations about sanitation elsewhere in the world than there were about conditions in the doctors' hometown. The Society urged Baltimore City to begin a diphtheria immunization campaign in 1932. In February, 1935, after the Baltimore City Health Department announced that it was discontinuing its home obstetrical services, the Society called for a study of maternal mortality in Baltimore. The first report was presented in December, 1936, and several additional years of study was recommended. As it turned out, before the study was wrapped up, more than 22 years of data were collected. The attack on Pearl Harbor in 1941 again shifted the attention of the Society away from domestic issues of public health and to the battlefront.

Another war occupied the proceedings of the Baltimore City Medical Society throughout the early post-war years: the war against socialized medicine. Public health issues receded as the national economy flourished throughout the Truman and Eisenhower administrations and government assumed more responsibility for community health. But in 1952, a Resolution was passed that supported the controversial fluoridation of the City's water supply:

> "WHEREAS, The Baltimore City Medical Society has always been interested in all fields of public health, and
>
> WHEREAS, it has been established under careful investigation that fluoridation of the city's water supply, one part to a million, is in nowise harmful, and
>
> WHEREAS, said fluoridation has been proved to be a definite preventive of tooth decay; therefore
>
> RESOLVED, that the Baltimore City Medical Society approves the fluoridation of the City of Baltimore water supply..."

"Have you ever heard of a thing called fluoridation? -- fluoridation of water? ... Do you realize that fluoridation is the most monstrously conceived and dangerous Communist plot we have ever had to face? ... A foreign substance is introduced into our precious bodily fluids without the knowledge of the individual ..."
-"General Jack Ripper"
in Stanley Kubrick's film Dr. Stangelove

On October 12, 1952, the Baltimore City Medical Society, with no reported discussion, unanimously passed a resolution urging Baltimore City to begin adding fluoride to the public water supply. As early as 1901, a Colorado Springs,

Colorado dentist, Dr. Frederick S. McKay, noted a brown stain on the teeth of some of his patients (indicating the condition called fluorosis) and that those patients seemed less susceptible to dental caries, which then could be treated only by extraction. In the 1930's, the National Institutes of Health conducted a study that collected data on the prevalence of childhood fluorosis and its inverse relationship to dental caries in 26 states. Yet as late as World War II, the main reason for selective service rejection was dental: Draftees who did not have a minimum of six opposing teeth were not eligible for the armed forces. By 1966, however, the incidence of dental caries among children who drank fluoride-treated public water had declined by over 68% since 1940. In 2000, over 1500 municipal water treatment systems incorporated fluoridation.

But as the fictional General Jack Ripper stated above, fluoridation was and remains controversial. After World War II, anti-fluoridation zealots claimed that the Nazi government used fluoride to make concentration camp prisoners docile before their murder. The Soviet government was reported to have imported fluoride from the U.S. for the same purpose in its GULAGS. American aluminum companies were accused of knowingly poisoning the population just to get rid of fluoride, a by-product of aluminum smelting.

When the Baltimore City Medical Society advocated fluoridation in 1952, they were also fighting a war against socialism and socialized medicine. While not labeling the Truman-era efforts to create a national health plan as "Commie plots," the politics of the Society were clearly very conservative. The Society recognized fluoridation for what it was, however: A classic example of clinical observation leading to epidemiologic investigation and community-based public health intervention. Millions of Baltimoreans were saved trips to the dentist and painful and disfiguring extractions while other cities debated the McCarthyite politics of fluoridation.

Yet the controversy continued into the 21st Century. The Fluoride Action Network, an advocacy group whose mission it is to end fluoridation of public water supplies worldwide, states that fluoride consumption is "ineffective and unnecessary," and links it to increased risk of arthritis, cancer, Alzheimer's Disease and hip fractures. It blames this "industrial waste product" for environmental disaster. The Leading Edge International Research Group calls fluoridation a conspiracy of the aluminum industry and government and compares its excesses to the Inquisition.

The only side effect to which fluoride's supporters admit is dental fluorosis. A wide body of scientific data concludes that fluorosis, while not cosmetically desirable, is otherwise harmless. Fluoride's supporters also agree that fluoride, consumed in excessive amounts is toxic. "Paracelsus knew it in the 1500s, when he set forth the principle that every substance is poisonous; the dose alone determines whether the substance will cause harm in a given situation," says William J. Bennetta of the California Academy of Sciences. Communist plot or public health boon? Ask your dentist.

Two years later the Society returned to a discussion that had twice before produced the same opinion of its members. The state Faculty passed on to the local organizations a proposal that a regional blood collection and distribution center be established in Baltimore by the American Red Cross. Only once, during the Korean War, had the Society approved such a move, and that was to be discontinued at the end of the conflict. Yet the Veterans Administration reported continuing difficulty in attracting adequate donors to meet its need for transfusions.

That the Society would object to the opening of an American Red Cross Blood Bank in Baltimore seems incongruous. Because the introduction of plasma during World War II made it possible to store material for a long period, the benefits of plasma had spawned blood banks across the country. But a close examination of the Society's letter shows that they did their homework and were addressing local availability of blood to civilians and veterans alike when they took a stand against the Red Cross proposal.

First, the Society's Blood Bank Advisory Committee pointed out that local civilian hospitals had no difficulty attracting donors. But that could change. "Since the Red Cross would plan to obtain 25,000 pints annually, this might well serve to disrupt the existing situation for civilian hospitals." Further, the Committee had polled the veterans' hospitals at Fort Howard and on Loch Raven Boulevard and at Perry Point and concluded that 400 pints monthly would be more than sufficient. So to open a blood bank that would seek to collect five times more blood than was actually needed represented a threat to the supply city-wide.

A practical plan was decided upon. The Committee recommended that the American Legion, perhaps in partnership with the Veterans of Foreign Wars, create a collection scheme that would enable the veterans' hospitals to tap the huge potential network of donors who were members of those organizations. The Committee also pointed out that the civilian fraternal organizations had excellent relations with central Maryland military posts, and that those stationed locally were excellent sources of blood donations, currently not being used by the veterans' hospitals.

The issue would not go away. In 1957 the American Red Cross again came to the Society, this time through the offices of a private citizen from the Baltimore Council of Churches, requesting the Society's backing in opening a civilian blood bank. This time, largely because of the testimony of Society Executive Board member Dr. John M.T. Finney, Jr., the decision was different. A motion was made to resurrect the Blood Bank Advisory Committee, but Dr. Finney pressed for a statement in support of the proposal immediately. He was not successful, and the Red Cross was advised that the "Baltimore City Medical Society heartily endorsed the idea of supplemental collections of blood and...had appointed a Committee to investigate the most efficient and economical manner of this supplemental collection." The Committee ultimately supported the new blood bank, which opened on December 1, 1958. "This is the culmination of a good deal of planning and effort," its final report stated. "We can all take genuine pride in our part in this development...The success...is now an accomplished fact."

During the late 1950's many less prominent items of public health advocacy were addressed. The Society wrote to City Hall asking that funds be found to add three extra trash collection days in 1959, as three summertime holidays were going to prevent trash pickup and the mounting piles of debris that would result were a health hazard. The Mayor was unable to finance three days of overtime for sanitation department employees and garbage steamed on Baltimore streets that summer. The same year, the Society, in response to a letter from the Motor Vehicle Administration, determined that new regulations for vision were advisable and that physical disabilities ought to be considered when drivers' licenses were issued. The recommendation was passed on to the state Faculty, as this was a statewide concern.

Public immunization goals were set, debated, and acted upon. This was an era of mass immunization, highlighted by the development by Dr. Jonas Salk of an anti-poliomyelitis vaccine. As early as February of 1956 a committee report was read into Society Minutes that described the Baltimore City Department of Education's plans to immunize the entire school population. The program "appeared to be designed to provide a means of making the vaccine available, but its execution provides no means of selection according to the ability to pay...It is more properly within the province of the Health Department to make available the vaccine to the indigent and within the province of the private physician to make available the vaccine to the private patients." The opinion was forwarded to Dr. Huntington Williams, Baltimore City Health Commissioner.

Pressured by the Medical and Chirurgical Faculty to support the school-based inoculation, in early 1957 the Society changed its mind and backed the program, as long as it was voluntary. A goal was set to have every citizen of Baltimore under the age of 40 vaccinated, but by mid-1959 the goal had not yet been met. Dr. Williams, accompanied by Dr. Robert E. Farber, Director of the city's Bureau of Communicable Disease, urged the Society to reverse its decision and support *mandatory* immunization. The Society's Executive Committee, in May, 1959, agreed and suggested to City Hall that immunization against poliomyelitis should be a condition of enrollment in any public school.

When mass immunization next appears in the Society's chronicles, the story is one of which "the Baltimore City Medical Society can be proud...for this project represents one of our main functions and that is to improve the general health of Baltimore." In early 1967, the "Measles Immunization Sunday" Committee was formed. The goal was to pick one day, and at various sites around Baltimore immunize as many children as possible. The Society's partners included its own Woman's Auxiliary, and the Baltimore City Chamber of Commerce.

Sunday, May 21, 1967 dawned bright, but the skies darkened and it began to drizzle early in the afternoon. It made little difference at the locations where volunteers from the Society were using the new inoculation guns as fast as they could pull the triggers. There were doctors furiously administering measles vaccine at each of the city's four health district offices, plus at Mondawmin Mall, where Dr. Ross Pierpont held sway and Reisterstown Plaza, where Dr. Roland Smoot headed a cadre of three volunteers. At the Montgomery Ward at Washington Boulevard and Monroe Street there were two volunteers hard at work, and past President Dr. D. Frank Kaltreider was on hand at Turner Armory near Hamilton. Recreation centers in Cherry Hill and Curtis Bay were manned by Society members, and Dr. John De Hoff, Baltimore's Assistant Commissioner of Health, was busy at the Druid Health Center.

When the lines finally ended at about 5:00 in the evening, a total of 14,420 children had been protected against measles. Children were inoculated at the rate of 2400 per hour, or four children per minute at each of the locations. For many of the physicians this was their first experience with the new inoculation guns, and at the program's headquarters, the office of Dr. Robert E. Farber, radio communications buzzed with requests for more vaccine and reports of gun failures all day long. But simply judging by the total of Baltimore children served, the day was a success. "We believe," Dr. Farber concluded, "in the future, we are going to have to rely on some sort of program similar to this...to meet the demands of our increasing population and great social change that is occurring."

The late 1960's and early 1970's found the Society concentrating on topics outside the arena of public health. Attendance at meetings dropped well into the lower double digits, not even enough for a quorum. A Civil Emergency Committee was formed after the 1968 riots in downtown Baltimore, but in general the attention of members was concentrated on medical economics and legislative matters.

When a Committee on Environmental Problems was convened in 1972 a new aspect of living in an urban center was addressed. The

Society had a long history of addressing smokestack issues, going back to 1907 when a Resolution was passed condemning the black smoke that hovered over Baltimore, and later when a noise ordinance was proposed. But nothing had ever been discussed in detail about the health ramifications of pollution, until, in 1973, Dr. Edward P. Radford, Professor of Environmental Medicine at Hopkins, addressed the membership. "Few...physicians are aware of the health hazards of pollution," the meeting announcement noted, "or what the role of the medical professional should be."

Gradually, the Society's direct involvement with issues of public health declined until, in 1986, the Committees on Public Health, Long Term Care and Environmental Problems were disbanded. Their functions were assumed by ad-hoc committees, to be created in the event a specific problem called for them, and to be closed upon solution of the problem. Meeting topics continued to address issues of public health, including drug addiction, care for the homeless and HIV/AIDS.

Baltimore City Health Commissioner Peter L. Beilinson, M.D. took the podium in the final decade of the Society's first century, with discussions such as his 1993 "Challenge of Improving Health Care in the City." Legislatively, Society members testified on public health issues such as handgun and firearm control and needle exchange, a program whereby intravenous drug users could exchange needles rather than passing them on, thereby reducing the transmission of HIV/AIDS. The annual "Stop Smoking Hotline" was inaugurated in 1994, and the following year fifty smokers called seeking advice on quitting the habit. Among the physicians taking calls was Dr. Susan Guarnieri, past Baltimore City Health Commissioner, and Dr. Beilenson, who was Commissioner at the time.

International terrorism invaded every aspect of American life after September 11, 2001. The anthrax attacks of October that year raised a new challenge to public health officials. Medical organizations could do little to prevent attacks, and technology was in place to effect a cure when treatment was timely. The Baltimore City Medical Society, following the lead of member Tyler Childs Cymet, D.O., wrote to members of the U.S. Congress in February, 2004, pointing out that victims of inhalation anthrax had been sick for over two years. "Who is responsible for the victims of terrorism?" it asked. A draft resolution prepared for the MedChi House of Delegates suggested that "...victims of an attack against the USA should be eligible for health care covered by the United States Government."

The days of yellow fever and malaria epidemics are long past, the diseases having been conquered due in part to the rigorous work of the renowned physicians who were members of the Baltimore City Medical Society. Constant advocacy in the early part of the century to clean the streets and the waterways, to provide healthy water and milk supplies and to make access to inoculation easy for everyone in Baltimore had accomplished the stated goals.

But this is not to say that the Society's role in improving public health had entirely disappeared. There were still challenges: Polluted drinking water may no longer have been a problem, but substance abuse was reaching deeper into Baltimore's increasingly poorer population. While maternal mortality had declined to respectable levels, family violence escalated.

During the twentieth century, the office of the Baltimore City Commissioner of Health and the Baltimore City Department of Health strengthened and became less politicized. Prior to 1900, Commissioners often served no longer than a one-year term (over 30 different physicians served in that position in the 1800s). In the 1900s, however, only eleven doctors held the post. Dr. Huntington Williams was Commissioner for 28 years.

This translated to a more pro-active and stronger Commissioner, altering the advocacy role of the Baltimore City Medical Society. Greater awareness of public health issues, coupled with increased levels of education and literacy among the general population, opened new opportunities for outreach that in part replaced earlier Society advocacy efforts.

Thus, the publication of the *BCMS Report*, a newsletter created by the BCMS Foundation to disseminate healthcare information directly to the consumers of same, became an important public health tool. *BCMS Report*, by advising patients of the necessity of flue vaccinations and by stressing the importance of breast self examination, among its many topics, became the Society's instrument of public health advocacy in an era when people had become better prepared to make their own healthcare decisions.

"Dr. Wm. J. Howard of Cleveland, Ohio, who had previously been invited by Dr. Cushing, read a most interesting paper upon 'The value of cooperation between medical, sociological and commercial organizations in the development of municipal hygiene and sanitation in Cleveland.' This was discussed by Drs. Wm.. H. Welch and Harvey Cushing...a considerable amount of enthusiasm was excited in connection with this subject..."

-Minutes, Baltimore City Medical Society
April 5, 1910

"CASE I. Mr. DeWitt arrived at his home after a journey of 4 or 5 days from N. Orleans. When he reached the depot he was curiously aphasic and unable to give directions of any kind...About 2 hours after I was sent for I found...heart sounds feeble and confused...perfectly conscious but could not articulate any account of his case and up to this time has no recollection of the exact date of his attack."

-Minutes of the Baltimore Medical Association
June 23, 1874

"Dr. Spratling read a very interesting paper on 'Epilepsy in the Young,' which was discussed by Drs. Gardner, Hunner and Spratling. Dr. W.S. Halsted gave a most instructive talk on the "General Consideration of the Treatment of Aneurism of the Large Arteries.' This was discussed by Drs. C. Urban Smith, and Halstead. Dr. D.R. Hooker read a paper on the so-called 'Sexual Necessity' and read numerous cards which had been received from the medical profession of the city relating to this subject. This paper was discussed by Drs. Pearce, Kintzing and Hooker."

-Minutes of the Baltimore City Medical Society
April 5, 1909

"Dr. Ulrich K. Henschke, Associate Professor of Clinical Radiology, Cornell University presented a discussion with several well-illustrated slides, depicting the treatment of otherwise untreatable malignancies by the use of interstitial radiation...Dr. Henschke pointed out that most of the cases he was given an opportunity to treat had previously been presented as candidates for radical surgery or conventional methods of external radiation...Dr. Henschke's talk was well received and was followed by a stimulating question and answer session by the members present."

-Minutes of the Baltimore City Medical Society
October 4, 1963

"By the frequent exchange of views...they may best promote the advance of medical science."

Scientific Sessions and Sections:
The Society's Role in Professional Education

Prior to the opening of the Maryland Medical College in 1807 (later the University of Maryland), physician education in Baltimore was mostly on-the-job-training. The earliest professional groups in the city and state were created largely to formalize medical education, establish proper venues for schooling, and certify students who, upon completing their education and passing an examination, were licensed.

The lack of a medical school in Maryland was noted nearly 20 years before Dr. Davidge opened the Maryland Medical College. "Philadelphia at this time furnishes the best school for Physic in America...Shall Maryland be insensible to the advantages of such an establishment?" wrote a correspondent to the *Maryland Journal and Baltimore Daily Advertiser* in June, 1790. It was, of course, possible to learn the trade, but it had to be done under the wing of a doctor who was willing to teach. The first such practitioner in Baltimore was Dr. Charles Friedrich Wiesenthal, who taught potential doctors from the rear of his residence at Gay and Fayette Streets and was instrumental in the founding of the city's first medical society. Behind his home and surgery he built a "dissection room," which faced Frederick Street. The dissection room was the scene of an attack in 1786 by an angry mob of righteous Baltimoreans that carried away the cadaver of an executed criminal that Dr. Wiesenthal was using in his anatomy instruction.

For most of their two centuries plus, medical societies served to fill the gaps in education offered in Baltimore. The earliest meeting Minutes surviving are of the Medico-Chirurgical Society of Baltimore, organized under the leadership of Dr. Samuel Baker in 1832. Their meetings include scientific and medical topics, and set the standard for medical societies to follow. On July 2, 1832, for example, they discussed whether or not Asiatic Cholera was contagious (two weeks later they decided that it was not.) Later that year Dr. John Fonerden asked in his talk "Does Neuralgia Depend upon Inflamation of Nervous Tissues?" Dr. Fonerden was the City Physician of Baltimore during the 1832 cholera epidemic and an early advocate of scientific care for the mentally handicapped.

In its 1866 Constitution, the Baltimore Medical Association listed as its first goal the "acquisition of knowledge." A Committee on

Lectures and Discussions was charged with the duty of selecting "members to lecture and propose subjects for discussion." Before normal business was conducted at a meeting there was to be the "Delivery of A Lecture or a Dissertation," followed by a discussion of the topic. Members then had an opportunity to present recent cases for the opinions and advice of their colleagues. Only after the scientific sessions did the Association turn to business.

While Minutes of the post-1904 Baltimore City Medical Society list only the topics covered during each meeting, accounts of patients, diagnoses and treatments covered in the nineteenth century societies' records offer a detailed look at medical practices. For example, on November 8, 1875, Dr. Taneyhill "exhibited a patient before the Association" whom he had been treating for epididymitis. The recording secretary, Dr. L.K. Merrick, noted the details of the case. The tumor had a "solid feel, commencing at the bottom of the scrotum....and would not permit light to pass through it." Following an accidental fall, the patient found that the tumor had completely disappeared. The Society proceeded to examine the patient, and Dr. Tiffany offered the opinion that the growth must have been gaseous. Dr. Noel recounted a patient he remembered with similar symptoms who was infected with syphilis. After he "drew off...clear fluid, which set up an inflammation that kept the man in bed for 10 days," a cure was effected. Dr. Philip C. Williams declared the entire case as much a moral as a medical question.

When attendance at Association meetings waned in the 1880's, and the question of what to do to encourage participation arose, some members felt that a strengthening of the science agenda was the answer, this being the principal mission of both the Association and the group that met in East Baltimore, the Medical and Surgical Society. In the end, the two organizations agreed to merge, and the newly formed group continued the medical and scientific sessions. In 1884, the Executive Committee requested that members write in advance of any subjects of particular interest, especially if the examination of a patient or a specimen was involved, so that these could be highlighted in meeting announcements.

When the American Medical Association mandated the reorganization of its state and local affiliates in 1904, the scientific and education agendas were organized into "sections." The new Baltimore City Medical Society adopted the national group's format, and announced the creation of sections covering Clinical Medicine, Pathology and Surgery, Obstetrics and Gynecology, Neurology and Psychiatry, Ophthalmology and Otology, Laryngology and Rhinology, and "as many sections as may at any time be proposed in writing by ten members." Each section was to nominate its own officers and conduct its own affairs, to report back to the general membership on a regular but unspecified schedule.

Additional sections were added as the need arose. The Medical Examiners Section, for instance, was not organized until 1910, when on the motion of Dr. W.E. Magruder, on behalf of 33 members who were interested in the section, it was formed. A section on dermatology was added in December, 1911 followed in 1920 by the Section of Roentgenology. Pediatricians got their section in 1934 and in 1937 the Orthopedic Club of Baltimore was admitted to the Society as an Orthopedic Section. Commonly, scientific sessions were listed as joint meetings with the Society general membership and a particular section, and often a guest speaker prepared a related topic. In 1925, for example, in a joint meeting with the Oto-Laryngological Section, Dr. William F. Moore of University Hospital in Philadelphia discussed "Etiology, Pathology and Bronchoscopic Treatment of Asthma."

The establishment of specialty sections marked a change in the way the Society handled its technical mission. Gone were the individual case studies that had aroused such intense discussions in the late 1800's. Scientific presentations continued, but moved from shop talk to broader clinical studies. Many topics addressed matters of public health - "The Importance of the Water Loan as a Public Health Measure" rather than "The case of a gentleman, age 50, who suffers from spells of vomiting," or of medical business - "The Economic Basis of Preventive Medicine" (1910) instead of "A successful case of tracheotomy for diphtheric croup" (1874). Epidemics captured the Society's attention, but discussions moved from the consideration of individual patients - "Mr. C, 30 years of age, had a mild attack of typhoid" (1883) - to citywide or statewide examinations of epidemics - "An analysis of the reports of cases of typhoid fever during the past four years" (1908).

Broader topics were covered, though the meeting agenda may still reflect a seemingly unrelated schedule of talks. On March 19, 1926 there were sessions on causes of failure in regional anaesthesia, carcinoma of the colon, recent advances in gynecology, and diagnosis and treatment of laryngeal tuberculosis. Frequency of meetings between 1904 and World War II varied from bi-weekly to monthly, but every meeting included at least 3 scientific topics.

Eventually, the scope of many talks in the scientific program widened even more: "Community Problems Relevant to the Problem of Alcoholism (1958), "Medical Care: The Consumer and the Provider" (1965), "Emotional Problems of Adolescence" (1968), "Caring for Opioid Dependent Intravenous Drug Users (1997), and

"Cancer: New Developments in Prevention and Control" (2002).

A Formal Approach to Professional Education

Baltimore City, with two important medical schools, was known internationally as a center of medical education, but the Baltimore City Medical Society recognized gaps in the post-graduate curricula for practitioners. As various societies had attempted to fill gaps in the past, by providing venues at which young physicians could learn from their more experienced colleagues and hear presentations made by academicians from distant universities, the Society in 1927 began to examine how it could provide for the post-graduate education of its members. A Committee to Study Facilities for Graduate Medical Teaching was established. In March of that year the Committee made its first report to the general membership:

> "The hospital situation in Baltimore...does not lend itself in any way to a general effort towards organized postgraduate teaching. With the exception of the two medical schools...no hospital attempts to have a routine attendance on the part of its clinical staff and in consequence no systematic teaching effort would be possible.
>
> Should it prove possible to organize a sufficient number of graduate courses in the various hospitals, the Baltimore City Medical Society might serve as a coordinating agency. An office might be maintained at which prospective students could receive information and be formally registered for the various courses. Such an office could also furnish to visiting physicians from the counties information in regard to the time and place of clinics and lectures in the various hospitals of the City."

The gap in postgraduate opportunities was filled in part by the Society, but not until 1963. That year, it was suggested that the Society seek accreditation from the American Academy of General Practice, and that its scientific sessions be considered as credit courses. Two goals would be accomplished by this: recognition of the value of the sessions presented by the Society by the Academy, and hopefully increased attendance at Society meetings. In 1964 an ambitious agenda of scientific topics was put forth, but there was no mention of credits to be granted. Finally, in 1965, the sessions on gastroenterology, featuring ten speakers, were approved for two hours of Category I credit by the Academy, and it was announced that the balance of the year's scientific agenda would also grant credits to participants.

Gradually, the focus of the professional education sessions moved from pure science to mix of medicine, administration and law. In 1972, after realizing that many patients do not understand their doctor's charges, especially in light of the confusing federal regulations, the Society produced a session on "Medicare Law." (In 1971, the Professional Relations Committee reported that of 122 complaints received that year, the vast majority were misunderstandings of fees). In 1973 a series of symposiums on the business of a medical practice was inaugurated. The following year the Society discussed the "Social Aspects of Medical Ethics", noting that ordained principles of medical ethics had not changed since 1803 while practical medicine - abortion, genetic engineering, organ transplants, and death and dying in particular - had advanced beyond the 170-year old precepts.

Throughout the 1980's and 1990's the Society offered Continuing Medical Education credit for the wide variety of courses on its curriculum. Meeting announcements reflected the changing environment in which physicians practiced: "Understanding your Difficult Patient," "Collective Bargaining/Unionism and Anti-Trust Laws," "Family Violence: Doctor, I Need Your Help!," and "The Alternative to Physician Assisted Suicide." While the organization struggled with falling membership and dues, it vowed to maintain its educational programs, often working with other local components of the state Faculty, with MedChi itself, and with the Monumental City Medical Society to sustain a relevant selection of courses.

Quarterly meetings continued and an active schedule of professional education evolved in the post-September 11 era. Peter Beilenson, M.D. returned in his capacity as Commissioner of the Baltimore City Department of Health to speak about bioterrorism in 2002 and the Society participated in a regional terrorism exercise early the next year. The occasional scientific topic was addressed, but as the modern Baltimore City Medical Society prepared to celebrate its centennial, a clear professional education mission had emerged. That mission, "...to advance the ethical practice of medicine and improve the quality of medical care by...providing advocacy and education programs..." had changed dramatically in its application in over a century.

"Two doctors cannot be together more than a few minutes before one of them says 'I had a case once...', and off they go."
-John B. De Hoff, M.D.
from a 2004 interview

"The following Fee Table was adopted at a meeting of the Medico-Chirurgical Society of Baltimore & other members of the profession in this city after much deliberation on each fee which it designates; And in no instance was a fee adopted without patiently enquiring - What is a just compensation to the Physician? What will intelligent Citizens consider to be just?"

- Medico-Chirurgical Society of Baltimore Minutes
March 4, 1833

"The Gentlemen of the Faculty in this town (of Baltimore) have suffered in respect to their bills...From the fluctuation of prices, and the unfixt value of money, they find it necessary to charge for their services in country produce or by way of barter."

-Dr. Andrew Wiesenthal
1799

The Baltimore City Medical Society and the Economics of Health Care

What has become a vexing and complicated issue for medical practitioners, political leaders and consumers of health care in the 21st century - the question of how to allocate the cost of medical services among the recipients, insurance companies, non-governmental bodies and government agencies that assume some of the responsibility for payment - is nothing new. How much should health care cost? Who should be responsible for paying the bill? How are those who provide it to be compensated for their education, their skills and their time? Dr. John De Hoff commented that until the end of World War II, most private physicians labored "on the edge of indigence." "My father," he recalled, "worked without a fee much of the time because that was what was expected of the family doctor." These questions have been discussed by every medical organization at every political level since medical societies were created.

During the first 100 years of the Baltimore City Medical Society, questions of the economics of medical practices occupied more time on the agenda than any other. It is a complex issue. It involves not only the compensation of the physician, but also influences the extent of a patient's access to a doctor's care and the means of that access, affects the physician's ability to control individual cases and ultimately determines to whom the physician is answerable. In general, the medical community has not been happy with the answers given by the various legislatures which make decisions on these things. The question of who is to pay for what remained unanswered as the Society entered its second century.

The professional opinion has generally hinged on the differentiation of medical care financing plans for those able and those unable to pay. Physicians' advocacy groups have generally favored government financing for the poor, although not always been without dissent, and leaving responsibility for those able to pay the premiums with private insurers. Progress towards the laudable goal of providing access to health care for everyone, regardless of social or economic class, has been slow and painful. But some progress has obviously been made. At least in the United States, few modern doctors must anticipate receiving payment in butter, eggs and live chickens.

As the modern Baltimore City Medical Society entered its second century in 2004, the largest federal health care program, Medicare, was "reformed", by a huge increase in the future pharmaceutical benefits to be provided by the massive entitlement. Like every other effort of Washington to address the problem of health care economics, this initiative was controversial. Opponents on both sides of the aisle claimed either that the new legislation was far too costly and transferred too burdensome a debt to future generations, or that the law did not go far enough in meeting the needs of lower income citizens, particularly in its centerpiece, provision for drug coverage. It was judged by the nation's largest advocacy group for the elderly to be a benefit worth enfranchising, and by others to be nothing short of a multi-billion dollar windfall for pharmaceutical and insurance companies. In all likelihood, it was a bit of all those things.

The notion of health insurance dates to the 16th century in Germany when guilds, small groups of skilled workers, negotiated the first of what would now be recognized as group hospitalization plans. It was even then equally a question of access to care as well as payment for that care. Before 1860, in both Europe and the United States, medical services were largely available only to the socially elite, provided by physicians working in exclusive private consulting rooms. In major cities there were outpatient clinics for the poor, manned by inexperienced doctors, medical students, and veteran doctors who chose to volunteer some of their time. Members of the Baltimore Medical Association, the Medical and Surgical Society of Baltimore and the Baltimore City Medical Society were among the attending, volunteer physicians at both the Baltimore General Dispensary and the Baltimore Almshouse.

By the late 1800's an increasingly better educated European working class was clamoring for more sophisticated medical care. Advances in surgery, in particular, fueled the demand for hospital services, and access by poorer patients with chronic diseases put pressure on a nation's medical resources. Often, the decision to operate in the case of a chronic disease like cancer was made based on financial criteria, as still only the well-to-do could afford conservative long-term care (long-term care being the more costly). Rapid progress in all aspects of health care, the public's access to information through an expanding media network, and industry's realization that the loss of wages was also a reduction of factory productivity all resulted in increasing demand for services.

Germany pioneered state-sponsored programs to provide financial protection in the case of illness and to pay for medical care, offering plans to industrial workers and their families in the late 1880s. Great Britain followed in 1911, creating a National Health Insurance program that replaced lost wages and paid for hospitalization for the working poor. The middle and upper classes were left to fend for themselves.

In Baltimore before the end of Word War I, physicians were beginning to examine the impacts of medical insurance, both private and government programs like those in Europe. In February, 1918, the Baltimore City Medical Society held a "symposium on the subject of health insurance." Dr. J. Hall Pleasants, Chairman of the Faculty Committee on Health Insurance, delivered an address entitled "Some Medical Aspects of Health Insurance." Sharing the podium with Dr. Pleasants was W. G. Curtis, Chairman of Education of the Insurance Economics Society of America.

Discussions of health insurance on a national level began in 1911, when the AMA established a committee to study the "sickness insurance" schemes that were then available in some European countries. In 1917, the AMA instructed its Council on Health and Public Instruction to "continue and make reports on the future development of social insurance legislation." The war intervened, and it was not until 1920 that a policy regarding public financing of health care was devised. It was straightforward in its opinion: "The American Medical Association declares its opposition to the institution of any plan embodying the system of compulsory contributory insurance against illness, or any other plan of compulsory insurance which provides for medical service to be rendered to contributors or their dependents, provided, controlled or regulated by any state or the federal government."

This remained the AMA's policy for many years. In 1922, the AMA House of Delegates repeated its opposition to all manner of government-sponsored coverage. That same year a proposal to provide group coverage for all AMA employees was tabled, and such coverage was not available to them for another two decades.

Though many of the working and middle classes were thrust upon the public's mercy during the Great Depression of the 1930's, little of the Depression's effects upon Baltimore is evident from the Minutes of the Baltimore City Medical Society. In December, 1932, the Society voted to send $300.00 of its $400.00 surplus to the Baltimore Relief Campaign. The Society's funds were supplemented by a $700.00 contribution from its members. This was the Society's only Depression-related contribution as a group. Undoubtedly, individual members stepped up their volunteer time and their talents, without collecting their fees, to help those from whom access to health care was taken by the Depression.

But while Society members were still attending meetings that were primarily scientific in nature, others in Baltimore were devising plans for hospitalization insurance. In March, 1934, Dr. Warfield T. Longcope, President of the Society, received a letter from Dr. Winford H. Smith.

> "I am writing to you as Chairman of the Baltimore Hospital Conference...As you know, the Baltimore Hospital Conference has presented to the hospitals of Baltimore a plan for the formation of an association known as the Baltimore Hospital Service Association; the purpose of which shall be to sell group hospitalization insurance to regularly employed persons of moderate means...The majority of all the general hospitals of the City have approved the plan, provided it meets with the approval of the Baltimore City Medical Society..."

A special meeting was called for April 13, 1934 to consider the report of the Society's Committee on Group Hospitalization Insurance. Unfortunately, the proceedings of the special meeting are lost, summarized by just three words: "Above Plan Rejected."

Nationally, the pros and cons of hospitalization coverage and government intervention in health care were being argued at all levels of professional organization. In theory, doctors should not object to a third party paying medical bills, be it a private insurer or a government agency. But in practice, physicians saw insurance as a threat to their autonomy, their privilege to charge fees that each thought represented fair remuneration, and ultimately the right to practice subject to the evaluation of their peers only, not a regulatory agency run by bureaucrats.

The greatest worry, however, was that physicians would gradually become employees of government and insurance companies. The third party payers would become the dispensaries of the future, depriving doctors of their traditional right to regulate themselves. In Europe, where the practice of public insurance policies had been in effect for several decades, insurance had spawned new competition from non-traditional sources like homeopathy as well as from doctors with abbreviated training. European medicine was seen by American doctors as being carried out based more on financial criteria than medical.

After rejecting the hospitalization plan put forth by the Baltimore Hospital Conference in 1934, the Society met to develop a plan of its own. On July 8, 1936, a special meeting was called to order to consider a plan proposed by the Medical-Dental Service Bureau, and agreement on a plan was reached:

> "Be it resolved...that a Group Hospitalization Plan similar to that inaugurated and operated by the Medical Societies and Hospitals in Washington, D.C. and St. Louis, Missouri, be inaugurated and put into operation promptly in Baltimore; that the members of this Society accept associate membership in the membership corporation to be formed, known as the Hospital Service of Baltimore, Incorporated."

The policy described at the 1936 meeting would be made available to breadwinners only (not to their family members, though that could be a future consideration). Employers that put together groups of ten or more insureds would deduct premiums from the employees' pay. Covered hospitalization was provided only upon the request of the insured's personal physician, and there was nothing to regulate the doctor's charge. Hospital bills, but not physicians' bills, were covered. Only "individuals in the low income group" were eligible, the determination to be made by the Medical-Dental Service Bureau, which was charged with administrative responsibilities. Board members of the new Group Hospital Service were nominated by the medical Society and hospitals.

The postcard announcing the special meeting had a second agenda item, a decision as to "the admission of colored physicians to the privileges of the Bureau." It was agreed that if the physicians were members of their national society they could be a part of the insurance plan. Curiously, the plan admitted all practicing white physicians, and they "did not necessarily have to belong to an organized City or State Society."

By October, 1936 the Medical-Dental Service Bureau was already a thousand dollars in debt, and a plea went out for more physician participation. Physicians were apparently content to vote in favor of the Society's plan but not to endorse it by their individual membership. The business community had, however, entirely bought into the plan, for the annual report of the Service Bureau closed by saying "The Bureau has received excellent cooperation from the industrial concerns of the city who wish this service available to their employees and, also, from the press. If the proper cooperation is given by the members of the Societies your Bureau will become a model for other communities to follow."

Within a year the Baltimore City Medical Society had soured completely on the insurance plan. In practice, the Hospital Service Corporation policy was covering doctors' bills in addition to hospitalization, something expressly forbidden by the Society. At the AMA Annual Meeting in 1936, a national precedent was set that differentiated physicians' and hospitals' charges in the pending Social Security legislation and the state and local organizations followed suit. Dr. Harvey Cushing, while not an AMA officer, was selected by the AMA to make its case in the White House. Dr. Cushing's daughter was married to President Roosevelt's oldest son. The original Social Security Act included only physician coverage for infant and maternal health and assistance for the blind and the physically handicapped, provisions which met with the AMA's approbation. Later, the AMA endorsed a private, voluntary plan that eventually became Blue Cross.

Based on the AMA Code of Ethics which prohibited third-party payment, either governmental or private, to "sell the services of practicing physicians on an annual premium basis," the Society in 1937 instructed its representatives on the Hospital Service Corporation Board to alter the Corporation's practice to conform with its code, and that of the AMA. There is little mention of the Corporation in subsequent meeting Minutes, but as late as 1941 the Society was still appointing members to serve on the Corporation's Board of Directors, so it can be assumed that the required changes to payment policy were made, and hospitalization only, not doctors' fees, was covered.

Nationally, the AMA found itself in court, in part over the issue of prepaid insurance coverage that included doctors' fees. While it had approved Blue Cross, the Association received warnings from the Justice Department of a potential indictment for monopolistic practices. The defendants, which included not only the AMA but also the Medical Society of the District of Columbia and the Harris County (Texas) Medical Society, were charged with denying membership to physicians participating in the Group Health Association of Washington, a pre-paid insurance plan. A guilty verdict was returned, and sustained over four years of appeals.

If physicians' groups sought to discourage their colleagues from honoring pre-paid plans to cover their charges, it may have been because they saw as the greater need the improvement of services in general rather than the expansion of access. This was highlighted by a nationwide study done in 1937 by the American Foundation of New York. Sixty Maryland doctors participated, including Baltimore City Medical Society president Dr. Warfield T. Longcope, and Society members Doctors Emil Novak, John M.T. Finney, Harry and Jonas Friedenwald, George Stickney, and others. As reported in the *Sun* in 1937, "Leading physicians and surgeons in the United States, consider that the medical profession's most pressing problem is improvement in the quality of medical care, rather than spreading the benefit of present medical knowledge to larger groups of people...The doctors know that costs are too high for the average income, and that there are all too many groups or regions in the country that certainly do not have adequate medical care...But even these things seem secondary to the pressing need to produce better medicine..."

The Wagner-Murray-Dingell Bill and Socialized Medicine

World War II interrupted discussion of such medical issues worldwide, but by 1943 the AMA was looking beyond the global conflict and at the face of medicine following war's end. Until then, the national Association had conducted limited public debate about health care financing, third party payment schemes, and the increasing challenges of meeting medicine's economic needs as technology made care more and more costly. Finally, the AMA determined that an office in Washington, DC was a necessity, with operations still controlled tightly from the Chicago headquarters. Emerging ideas about what the Association called "socialized medicine", in particular the Wagner-Murray-Dingell Bill of 1943 and President Truman's 1945 health care financing proposals, both of which called for an American version of national health care insurance, caused the AMA to look again at the strength of its lobbying program. The issue of physician and hospital reimbursement, however, still faced decades of controversy.

Locally, the Baltimore City Medical Society was equally concerned about the implications of social legislation. The group went on record against the Wagner-Murray-Dingell Bill predicting that passage would "inevitably lower the quality of medical care given to the American public, and seriously endanger our presently high level of health..." More than that, the Bill, if passed, was accused of "destroying our 'Freedom of Enterprise Concept'," and would "sacrifice Free Enterprise principles in the distribution of medical care in the United States." The Society voted to oppose the Bill, in line with the decision of the AMA.

But the spectre of a federally-mandated pre-payment plan, for the poor as well as for those capable of paying for private insurance, failed to disappear. The Society met in 1948 to consider a proposal to support the Maryland Medical Service Plan, hoping that Washington would step back if every state adopted a system to pay the total medical costs for the lower income class, and provide limited benefits for other income classes. President John T. King, M.D. opened a special meeting on March 24, 1948 with a brief history of the Plan, which unfortunately was not detailed in the Minutes. It brought about immediate and lively debate. Some members wanted to oppose the plan entirely without proposing any alternatives. Others, after learning that 38 other states had already instituted similar pre-payment programs, concluded that broad-reaching medical insurance, with some government regulation, was inevitable and that a proactive course would be best. It appears as if the majority of members at the meeting concurred that some sort of plan was needed for Maryland. In the end, a motion was carried that the Society "go on record as in favor of a plan. Period."

THE *Voluntary* WAY IS THE AMERICAN WAY
50 Questions You Want Answered on COMPULSORY
HEALTH INSURANCE Versus *Health...The American Way*

-Slogan and title from a 1945 American Medical Association brochure
"Wagner-Murray-Dingell and the 'Socialization' of Medicine"

Though the first Wagner-Murray-Dingell Bill never came to a vote, it elicited millions of words of both support and opposition. Introduced in the 1943 Congressional session, the Bill would have created a national fund from which medical care and hospitalization expenses were to be paid for each insured and the insured's family. Unlimited doctors' bills were included, as well as up to 30 days of hospitalization. Patients would be free to choose their physician from any who participated in the plan. Physicians only had to meet the cursory standards of the Surgeon General to be included. The bills were to be paid by a 1 1/2% employee deduction, matched equally by the employer.

Polls indicated that 74% of the population favored some form of national health insurance, and 68% believed that it should be a part of Social Security. In spite of public opinion, the reaction of the professional medical community was swift and decisive. It was suggested that government would limit the number of hours a physician could work daily, creating huge queues for care. Naysayers claimed that patients would be forced to go to doctors chosen by bureaucrats. Nationally, physicians' groups and drug companies spent over $250,000 - a huge sum in 1943 - to encourage the public to speak out against passage. The AMA established a Washington office, and contacted 8,000 community organizations, distributed anti-Truman legislation literature at over 9,000 libraries, reached 130,000 druggists and dentists and over 13,000 chambers of commerce. Even Congress could not turn a deaf ear to a campaign on that scale.

Support by organized labor and farm organizations was not enough to bring the Bill out of committee. Some would have liked it to cover the entire population rather then only those working (other government programs were proposed to provide services to the unemployed). Those critics pointed out that the Bill included nothing to encourage preventive health services and failed to induce physicians to join together in more effective group practices.

On November 19, 1945, President Truman again urged Congress to turn its attention to national health legislation. He sought a Bill which would increase grants to states for maternal and pediatric care, provide funds for hospital construction, and support medical education. Most important, he called for the expansion of Social Security to cover medical care, hospitalization, nursing, laboratory costs and dentistry. He also asked that the Bill provide for lost wages due to sickness or disability. Congressmen Wagner, Murray and Dingell altered their original Bill to meet many of these goals, but it was defeated in 1945, again in 1947, and finally laid to rest in 1949.

The Bill was first discussed at the Baltimore City Medical Society in October, 1945. As the final vote on Wagner-Murray-Dingell was reaching the House floor, the Society prepared a resolution which stated succinctly that it "does hereby go on record against any form of compulsory health insurance or any system of political medicine designed for national Bureaucratic control."

If the resolution were meant to be the Society's final word on "socialized medicine," it failed. The 1970's brought a tidal wave of ideas about public financing of all or parts of the nation's health care community, and the Baltimore City Medical Society, in concert with the Medical and Chirurgical Faculty and the American Medical Association spoke definitively about the changing role of government in medicine.

A questionnaire was sent out to each member about the advisability of devising some means of pre-payment insurance for the lower working and middle classes of Baltimoreans. Dr. W. Houston Toulson, who drew the responsibility of having to create a questionnaire that adequately explained the options and was, in its wording, non-partisan, presented the results. "It is difficult to prepare a report on the comments sent in; some wanted full benefits, some felt that full benefits were not workable; some were for a lower income level; some for a higher income level; some wanted hospital as well as house service, etc., etc."

Over half of the membership returned their completed questionnaires, a high level that indicates both interest and concern. The vote tally revealed that 80% of those polled were in favor of some sort of insurance plan. There were many comments. Whatever was decided, it should be called a "Non-Medical Service Plan" as it did not cover the cost of the practitioner. Radiologists complained that certain specialists were left out entirely. Arguments ensued about whether the majority of local doctors saw the need for a plan or not. Parliamentary rules were unsuccessfully called into question as a tactic to delay a decision by the Society. In the end, the following motion was carried:

"That the Baltimore City Medical Society instruct its delegates to the House of Delegates of the Medical and Chirurgical Faculty to request that a large committee, representing the City and County Societies, each hospital, representatives from each of the specialty groups and the general practitioners, be appointed to further study a possible medical service plan before any plan is adopted and that this plan be presented back to each of the various medical societies before any plan is adopted."

In spite of the growth of Blue Cross, the AMA preferred medical insurance carrier, legislation that would have enacted nationwide health insurance plans rose, and died, in the halls of Congress. Dr. John M.T. Finney, recently returned from a trip to England in February, 1949, reported to the assembled members of the Society on the state of medical affairs in England after the passage of that country's revised National Health Insurance act, which covered every citizen. "General Practitioners are having too few or too many patients. The cost of the program for the first year will be approximately twice that originally estimated."

Based on Dr. Finney's observations, a strongly-worded resolution firmly against any sort of federal government sponsored, mandatory health coverage was drafted by the Baltimore City Medical Society, signed by its president, Dr. Albert E. Goldstein on March 29, 1949, and sent to the White House. Wagner-Murray-Dingell was again in the Congressional Record. "WHEREAS, the experience of all countries where government has assumed complete control of medical services has shown that there has been...a progressive deterioration of medical standards and medical care to the detriment of the health of the people," the Society Resolution claimed. Maryland Senators and Congressman were "respectfully requested to use every effort at their command to prevent the enactment of such legislation."

The Truman administration was not willing to abandon one of its prized proposals, and in early December, 1950, President Truman again pledged to press ahead with his plans for a government-sponsored plan for everyone, whether elderly, employed or unemployed. Dr. Amos R. Koontz was the Chairman of the Baltimore City Medical Society's Committee on Public Medical Education. While the Committee had been formed for a variety of educational purposes, during the early 1950s it served principally as a vehicle to urge the public to write to their Federal legislators to object to the Truman plan. Dr. Koontz sent a letter to every member on December 4, 1950, warning them that without an immediate contribution, and monthly pledges to follow, the Administration would be successful. "This is an S.O.S. The treasury of the Committee on Public Medical Education in your fight against socialized medicine is bare - literally!"

Dr. Louis A.M. Krause was the President of the Society during the waning years of the Truman administration, and he was as dedicated to the defeat of what the White House had begun calling "National Health Insurance" as was Dr. Koontz. "...We cannot afford to lose sight of Congressional manoeuvres relating to health," he wrote to members. "There are a hundred different jobs that we can do to help. Apathy defeated France in 1940. Apathy has left us holding the bag on both military and civilian defense in this darkest period of our history.* Apathy can very well lead all of us to 'doctoring' for the Government under Federal directives and at Government pay."

Once again the combined force of most medical organizations in the nation stalled the Truman initiative. Another Wagner-Murray-Dingell Bill did not emerge from Congressional committees and the pressure for a national plan melted away in the economically favorable decade of the 1950s.

During the years of the Eisenhower administration, from 1953 until 1960, medical societies gained a respite from continual legislative activity. A few trial balloons were floated in Washington, one in particular sponsored by a young Senator from Massachusetts, John Fitzgerald Kennedy, had the support of the AFL-CIO and other labor organizations but went nowhere. The AMA decided to strengthen its advocacy wing by forming a political action committee, AMPAC in 1961. In 1965, during the first major challenge faced by AMPAC, the Committee's Chairman, Frank Coleman, M.D., laid out a clear agenda: "The solution to keeping politics out of medicine no longer lies in asking Congress to act wisely; the solution lies in helping to elect a wise Congress." But as well-placed as the national organization was to mount a defense against the centerpiece of Lyndon Johnson's Great Society initiative, Medicare and Medicaid, its lobbying efforts proved no match for the ex-Congressman from Texas in the White House.

Johnson's predecessor, John F. Kennedy, had added the power of the Executive to efforts to pass the King-Anderson Bill in 1961. The Society objected in a strongly-worded Resolution cast in March, 1962. "...there is no need for hasty and ill-conceived action in the passage of additional legislation...to provide a partial program of medical care for all those receiving Social Security payments...BE IT THEREFORE RESOLVED, that the Baltimore City Medical Society rejects any legislation providing medical care under the

---

*Probably refers to the McCarthy hearings and the "Red" scare

Social Security mechanism." King-Anderson would have provided medical care for all seniors, but the Bill was defeated in 1962 and the assassination in Dallas in November, 1963 put a temporary hold on medical legislation as well as many other government initiatives. The Johnson landslide in 1964, in retrospect, assured Medicare's passage, though the medical professional community failed to recognize the inevitability of Johnson's "Great Society" agenda. The AMA countered Medicare with Eldercare, a program which would have provided coverage for the needy elderly, but there was never any real hope that anything but a Johnson Bill would become law in a Congress and Senate heavily dominated by Democrats.

The debate over Medicare and Medicaid caused a rift between the Baltimore City Medical Society and the Medical and Chirurgical Faculty. MedChi approved a campaign to raise $140,000 to fight the passage of the Bills, and voted to fund the campaign by assessing each member $50.00. It was billed as a "continuing education campaign," ostensibly to inform the public about a wide range of medical matters, but as originally outlined, any physician who failed to participate financially was to have been denied his or her access to the state Faculty's Physician Defense Fund. Under vehement protestation, that clause was stricken, but doctors were threatened that if they did not pay the assessment by the end of 1965 they would be dropped from the membership roles, which had the same effect inasmuch as it ended the physicians' malpractice coverage.

"A tumultuous special session" is how the *Sun* billed the state Faculty's February, 1965 meeting to determine a course of action to fight Medicare. AMA President Donavan F. Ward, M.D. gave a prepared address comparing Medicare with the Association's Eldercare proposal. Three days later, the Faculty told a *Sun* reporter that it expected all local doctors to contribute to the "war chest."

This proved to be neither the last nor the most tumultuous gathering of physicians on the topic of the war chest. At a general meeting of the Baltimore City Medical Society in late March, at which the issue of the special assessment was not even on the agenda, the Society decided by a mere six votes to go along with the plan. There were only 90 members present. Three weeks later a special meeting was called with the assessment, and the Society's policy regarding Medicare, as the only agenda items. Three hundred physicians trooped to Cathedral Street this time, a standing room only crowd. In 1965, membership in the state Faculty amounted to about 2,800 practitioners. Fifteen hundred practiced in Baltimore City.

Ninety percent of those present voted against the levy. Dr. Helen Taussig, Society member and co-developer of the famous blue baby surgery, pointed out that it was "a very dangerous thing for a scientific society to...spend money on our image. If we do right, our image will take care of itself." A resolution was overwhelmingly passed asking the state Faculty to rescind the assessment.

No action was taken at the state level to repeal the decision. In August, 1965, the Faculty revealed that it had been requested to endorse a plan for physicians to individually boycott Medicare, which had been signed into law the previous month. Members had a right to "refuse to sign any papers...execute any certificate...or accept any fees from an agency of the United States government," it asserted. "Medicare will unquestionably lead to a deterioration of the present high quality, first class medical care," it went on to say. The state's policy was in lock-step with that of the AMA, in spite of the fact that AMA President Dr. Ward stated emphatically at the February MedChi meeting that "I did not make any statement that the AMA would strike or that doctors would strike. Let there be no misunderstanding that the doctors on the AMA level are contemplating any such thing."

Money was not the only criteria for the Society's decision to reject the special $50 assessment. Many Society members agreed with Frederick County physician Louis Schoolman, who equated the $140,000 to be raised as little more than something to line the pockets of an advertising agency. "Ten years of negativity has worn us out," he moaned. "Medicare will pass, and it becomes us to accept it in a dignified fashion." In a September letter to the membership of the Baltimore City Medical Society members, President Samuel Morrison, M.D., called upon members to recognize the changing times. "For a group which meets the public so intimately, it would appear that many of us have lost the common touch. Many are so haughty and righteous that they arouse indignation...we often appear not to reflect public opinion in the socio-political-economic spheres." The Society announced that Dr. Ivan L. Bennett, a Hopkins professor who had delivered a scathing attack on AMA policies at a medical school graduation earlier in 1965, would be the keynote speaker at its October general meeting.

On July 30, 1965, President Johnson signed the Medicare and Medicaid Bill (Title XVIII and Title XIX of the Social Security Act) in Independence, Missouri (the home of President Truman). Medicare provided health insurance for senior citizens, Medicaid financed medical care for the poor. Former President Harry Truman was on the dais with LBJ, who said "We marvel not simply at the passage of this Bill but that it took so many years to pass it."

The signal to the AMA and its component organizations was to learn to live with the federal government as a major part of the national health care delivery system, and the Baltimore City Medical Society, rather than lick its wounds and refuse to cooperate, turned its attention to things about which it could do something positive. The incoming President in 1970, Dr. John N. "Jake" Classen, said "the most pressing problems facing the Society are peer review and continuing medical education." Much of what would evolve in the peer review process involved mediating disputes between insurance companies, including Medicare and Medicaid, and practitioners. But the days of speaking out volubly against the extension of health care coverage sponsored entirely or in part by government agencies, in Annapolis and especially in Washington, were over.

What the AMA and others predicted would result should President Johnson's plans become law, given the hindsight of many years turned out to be true. Small practices became deluged in paperwork, and as early as July, 1966 complaints about the administrative burden began to appear in Society publications. Senator J. Glenn Beall, Jr. addressed the Society in March, 1972. "Washington is where the action is regarding legislation on health care delivery," the meeting announcement said. "Changes in Medicare and Medicaid laws...are being made this year and the Congress will consider national health insurance in the near future. Senator Beall will inform us of his views on these monumental topics."

The rise of Health Maintenance Organizations was discussed in 1974. The Education agenda changed gradually, incorporating more business-related topics that were geared toward helping physicians organize their offices around the demands of insurance billing procedures. Attempts were made to standardize billing forms, in an effort to simplify what was becoming a welter of varying demands from third-party payers, all of which delayed a doctor's compensation for service provided. A "Mini Course for Medical Secretaries" in 1976 taught skills in discussing insurance coverage with patients, rules for billing systems, credit and the law, and finally collection of past due bills. The course was repeated often as demand for it grew.

"The Blues" and the Rise of Private Medical Insurance

Almost 40 years before Presidents Truman and Johnson announced the formation of the country's first nationwide government-sponsored insurance plan, the groundwork was laid for what has since become the nation's largest private health care insurer: "The Blues." In 1929, Baylor University in Dallas, Texas created a group health plan for Dallas public schoolteachers that guaranteed 21 days of paid hospital care for a premium of $6.00/year. Other groups of Dallas working people learned of the program and were anxious to join. From these beginnings, Blue Cross began to quickly spread beyond the borders of the Lone Star State. Because Blue Cross expanded by establishing locally-operated insurance plans rather than maintaining a centralized management structure, it was gradually accepted by the medical community.

In 1938 a conference on national medical care economics was convened in Washington, and the American Hospital Association endorsed Blue Cross, adopting the official Blue Cross symbol as an indication that an individual plan met with its approval. With the Great Depression raging, there was pressure on Congress to do something to provide for a payment mechanism for health care, and in doing so to widen access to care. Both the AHA and the AMA were anxious to avoid the establishment of "socialized medicine," and the success of the Blues looked like an answer. So the following year, the AMA also approved pre-paid hospitalization insurance (as long as it did not include payment to individual practitioners), citing Blue Cross as an example of an acceptable plan.

The second "Blue", Blue Shield, was devised to provide medical care (not limited to hospitalization) to miners and lumbermen in the American northwest shortly after the dawn of the twentieth century. Both industries were booming and hugely profitable, both were labor-intensive and hazardous, and demand for workers exceeded supply. As was often the case, the improved access to medical care was provided to employees not because the companies were particularly charitable, but because management recognized the effect that worker loss due to injury had on the bottom line. Employers paid monthly premiums to medical "service bureaus," which were small groups of physicians formed to offer the pre-paid coverage and care. In 1939, what became the national Blue Shield system was founded in California when these small groups joined forces. The two Blues merged in 1982.

For three decades, the AMA and its local affiliates used Blue Cross and Blue Shield as a tool to forestall the implementation of a government-sponsored medical insurance plan. By and large, only working Americans were covered by the Blues, though coverage was slowly expanded to include an employee's dependents. Those who were retired, who were temporarily unemployed or permanently unemployable, or who simply had no job which provided group coverage were left uninsured. Provisions for providing and paying for medical care for the elderly and the indigent became the major battlefront in health care financing, and led ultimately to the adoption of Medicare and Medicaid. Medical organizations begrudgingly accepted Blue Cross and other similar plans for working Americans, maintaining all the while that the charitable efforts of their members, hospitals and state and local governments took care of those who had no access to private insurance. The only recourse for this substantial part of the population was the waiting line at the Baltimore General Dispensary, City Hospital and, after 1947, a bed at one of the hospitals that participated in the Baltimore City Health Plan; the only recourse, that is, until the 1965 passage of Medicare and Medicaid.

Medicare changed the way the nation would allocate and pay for medical care for the elderly, but Medicaid had an equal impact on American society's philosophy regarding care for the poor and the indigent. Access to health care was, and still is, as much a function of economics as of logistics. The question from the earliest days has always been "Who will pay the caregiver?" In the case of medical attention for the lower classes, the answer has usually been charity, or in recent times, a combination of free clinics and the government.

Until 1965, the responsibility rested on the shoulders of private charitable organizations, the generosity of private doctors who volunteered their time, and state and local government. Baltimore's earliest charity of the sort, the Baltimore General Dispensary, continued to offer services to those unable to pay for them until 1959, its 158th year. The Almshouse, on Calverton Street in far west Baltimore, originally designed as a depository for the poor, also offered medical care (often the best available in the city, as its wealth of interesting cases drew the attention of the finest medical students in Baltimore, as well as some of the city's most progressive physicians). In 1802, Dr. James Smith, who was the attending physician at the Baltimore County Almshouse, established a Vaccination Institution in the city to innoculate the poor against smallpox. By 1812, 38 members of the Medical and Chirurgical Faculty, a large percentage of whom were also active in Baltimore medical societies, were volunteering to vaccinate any citizen who applied, free of charge.

"That all fines imposed in Baltimore County on persons convicted of keeping houses of ill fame shall be and are hereby appropriated to the use of the said General Dispensary..."
-from the original charter of the Baltimore General Dispensary
1801

The Indian Queen Tavern, corner of Baltimore and Hanover Streets, was one of Baltimore's most prestigious hostelries when, in February, 1801 a group of 12 concerned citizens gathered under its smoke-blackened beams to devise a plan for caring for the poor citizens of the city. When they completed the draft of the Charter of the Baltimore General Dispensary (including the curious source of funds cited above) they had created one of the nation's earliest charities devoted to the medical care of the poor.

THE BALTIMORE CITY MEDICAL SOCIETY - A History

Within a year, 10 physicians were assigned to various Baltimore wards, at a salary of $300/year, which was moderate at best for a doctor. Many other attending physicians received no pay at all. Those who wished to send poor patients to the Dispensary could do so, after paying an annual fee of $5.00. There were never enough funds to meet all the demands placed upon the Dispensary, however, even in 1809 when the Sheriff of Baltimore County sent $85, the total of fines collected from the operators of "houses of ill fame."

During the 158 years the Dispensary's doors were open to the needy, 950,310 patients were treated and 1,569,311 prescriptions were filled. In that span about 170 doctors generously volunteered their time, or accepted pay well below what their private practice yielded. But by 1959 it became apparent that other mechanisms for treating the destitute were working well, and a decision was made to establish a foundation through which the Dispensary's assets could be managed and a wider variety of charities supported. The Dispensary's last home, at the corner of Paca and Fayette Streets, still bears the proud name BALTIMORE GENERAL DISPENSARY in its stonework.

Many of the physicians associated with the Dispensary were active members of local medical societies. Dr. Samuel Baker, founder of the Medico-Chirurgical Society of Baltimore, was an attending physician there. Dr. John Beale Davidge, founder of what became the University of Maryland Medical School, was one of the Dispensary's first attending physicians. The founder of the Society for the Promotion of Vaccination, Dr. James Smith, was an early attending physician. Dr. Isaac E. Atkinson, a President of the Baltimore Medical Association, was an attending physician at the Dispensary. Of the 8 physicians who founded the Baltimore Medical Association in 1866, 4 had been vaccination physicians, who during times of epidemics provided vaccinations to the needy at no charge. Dr. Robert Parke Bay, who was President of the Baltimore City Medical Society in the 1930s served on the Dispensary's Board of Managers.

Many of those whose names do not appear in the Dispensary's history were serving elsewhere. Dr. Louis McLane Tiffany President of both the Baltimore Medical Association and the state Faculty, was a visiting physician at the Baltimore Almshouse. The Almshouse was established in 1773 to care for those incapacitated by disease, physical handicaps, old age or otherwise incapable of providing for themselves. The Almshouse, unlike other institutions, admitted free blacks and would treat slaves at the owner's expense (The Baltimore General Dispensary refused service to "any bondservant or slave, or to any other person who may be considered competent to the payment of a physician.")

Until the passage of Medicaid in 1965, charities like these two, plus dozens of others, provided the bulk of medical care to Baltimore's needy. Most of the staff, for nearly two centuries, consisted of hundreds of volunteers or practitioners willing to work for a small fraction of their normal fee.

After reorganization in 1904, the Baltimore City Medical Society regularly, though not frequently, discussed the plight of the city's poor residents, the best way to bring medical services to blighted neighborhoods and to meet the challenges of health care needs associated with poverty. While the Society always took the moral high road, and while many of its members continued to offer their services voluntarily at the various institutions that served the poor, the attitude developed that the lower class was the responsibility of local government. In 1911, after being convinced by a presentation by Dr. Standish McCleary that the treatment of alcoholics in the city was ineffective at best, the Society formed a committee to study the possibility of establishing a city-operated "farm" for alcoholics. A connection between alcoholism and poverty was made in the discussions that led to the motion. A month later the committee was discharged without having made any recommendations, responsibility for future discussions devolving to the state faculty.

Throughout its pre-Medicaid history, accounts of Baltimore City Medical Society proceedings report the group's concern with inadequate beds at Baltimore City Hospitals and the Sydenham Hospital for Contagious Diseases, creation of a blood bank to provide blood to the indigent at no charge, work with the Red Cross, and the city's plans to provide medical care for "families on relief." In 1953, the Society, under the leadership of Dr. J. Wesley Edel, considered a proposal to formally discount doctors' fees, on a standardized basis determined by the patient's ability to pay. The Baltimore *Sun* reported that "Dr. Edel has proposed the plan to ease the cost of private medical care for lower income groups and thereby eliminate any possible need for socialized medicine in this country."

Other members had a different perspective, however, and on January 12, 1953 the headline read "Doctors Veto Plan for Fee Cooperative." A five-man committee appointed by the Society spent less than 3 months examining the Edel program. Under the plan, patients were to register with a Cooperative to be supervised by the Society. Physician participants would have paid five dollars annually, and clients one dollar. Clients would carry membership cards that identified their discount class, and all participating doctors would agree to accept the card. The benefits were only good for physician and surgeon care, not hospitalization, pharmaceutical products, or non-approved therapies.

The Committee rejected the plan for several reasons. The most important was that they felt there was no health care crisis among the poor of Baltimore. Patients reported that they could already receive discounts if they only asked for them. The Committee also objected to the label of "indigent" that may be inappropriately applied to otherwise upstanding citizens. It violated the principal of personal care as well. "The plan is very impersonal. [The] patient-physician relationship is jealously guarded and is excellent at this time." Finally, and in retrospect an especially prophetic observation, it would "increase paperwork."

On a statewide level, the Medical and Chirurgical Faculty had been working with the State Department of Health for ten years on a practical plan to care for the state's poor. Despite the contentions of local societies that adequate care was already being provided on a charitable basis, a report drawn by the Committee of Medical Care of the Maryland State Planning Commission, on which MedChi members served, recognized in 1943 that "...although Maryland is fortunate in her wealth of medical facilities and the general high level of medical care which her citizens receive and although the medical profession on a voluntary basis unselfishly and untiringly renders medical care to the medically indigent, certain important deficiencies exist." The deficiencies came down to the observation that in certain parts of the state, essential medical services were simply unavailable to the poor.

A plan grew out of the committee report which provided for care for residents of Maryland's 23 counties, but not Baltimore City. "Establishing a Bureau of Medical Care in Baltimore City was not included...because it represents a far more complex problem and will be made the subject of a separate study." The State Board of Health approved the plan and in the 1945 legislative session in Annapolis it was adopted. In his announcement, Governor Herbert R. O'Conor said "As one who has unbounded confidence in the integrity of the medical profession, I am opposed to Socialized Medicine as I believe that the adoption by Maryland of the program proposed would make unnecessary the entrance of the Federal Government into the field of medicine in this State."

Two years later a similar plan was put into action in Baltimore City. Organization was radically different than the state plan because of the presence of "two great medical schools and their hospitals" in the city. "The eventual success of the Baltimore Health Plan...may revolutionize the social functions of the hospital and its relationship to the community." The plan was presented to the Baltimore City Medical Society at a special meeting in December, 1946 by the Chairman of the Committee on Medical Care of the Maryland State Planning Commission, Dr. Maurice C. Pincoffs. The following October a Resolution was approved "that the Baltimore City Medical Society is in favor of this new work being undertaken in Baltimore in a comprehensive manner...and urges the physicians of Baltimore to cooperate with the Commissioner of Health in making the new work successful in the best interests of the people."

As a group, the Baltimore City Medical Society continued to consider the various Bills that passed through local and state legislatures regarding health care for the poor, and on occasion mounted campaigns to provide that care. After the introduction of the Salk vaccine in the mid-1950's, the Society eventually advocated for city-wide inoculation of school children, at no cost. A short-lived program to provide medical care for those recently-unemployed during the economic slowdown of the 1970's served many unfortunate Baltimoreans, and was disbanded when the economy turned around. The Society worked to establish a free blood bank for the indigent in 1977. Members continued, individually, to volunteer at city clinics.

An altogether different insurance issue, however, eventually prevented Society members from participating in some charity programs. For many years, Society members, at no charge, provided brief examinations for incoming Boy Scouts at the Broad Creek camp in Harford County, certifying that each boy was physically capable of participating in scouting activities. A proposal to enlist volunteer doctors to provide care for the homeless began in 1989. Both of these programs were discontinued by the Society because of the looming threat of malpractice litigation.

The First Professional Liability Crisis

Though the Society failed to mention its establishment, a Physicians Defense Fund was in place by 1933 to help a member defray the cost of defending himself against malpractice charges. An April, 1933 change to the by-laws made it clear that "Only members paying their dues prior to January 31st are eligible for Physicians' Defense." None of the early Treasurer's Reports note a balance in the fund (as there is no balance sheet presented at all), nor do they account for money coming into the fund.

The fund, however, to the extent that it functioned at all represents the Society's first effort toward providing financial support for members who faced malpractice suits. Also in 1933, Dr. Charles Brack outlined a malpractice policy offered by Aetna Insurance Company. "Whereby if fifteen men take out insurance against malpractice the premium will be reduced from twenty-five dollars to eighteen dollars." Other economic issues dominated the work of the Society's legislative committee, and malpractice did not arise as a serious threat until 1956.

That year, Society counsel G.C. Anderson, reported a "tremendous increase in the number of malpractice suits throughout the country, as well as the increase in the amount of settlements, and pointed out that they were increasing in Maryland as well." Mr. Anderson was concerned that he could not properly defend against these charges without the cooperation of a panel of expert witnesses. Because an expert witness could expect to spend several days in court and away from his practice, the panels had failed to materialize when needed. One week after speaking to the Executive Committee, Mr. Anderson made his plea to the membership, asking for the election of a panel that could be depended upon to consult and when necessary, testify. Premiums do not seem to be at issue in 1956, only culpability.

Physician liability became a more important issue for the Society and its members, and in 1975 the issue moved to Annapolis and the struggle to find a plan that would satisfy everyone - physicians, patients and attorneys alike - began in earnest. "Malpractice is the big word...in Annapolis this year," the February Newsletter announced. That year, a Bill to establish a Medical Injury Compensation Commission was written, but not approved. The Bill would have created a 3-man commission to study every case, set a limit on dollar amounts which could be awarded as well as a limit on attorneys' fees. As might have been expected, the trial lawyers objected. The goal of the physicians was to improve the insurance climate in Maryland, as even this early professional liability coverage had become a seller's market. Insurers had threatened to leave Maryland on April 30th if a consensus was not achieved.

While legislation was not passed, a Special Committee to Study Malpractice was formed and early indications were that an arrangement of binding arbitration, based on the opinion of a committee nominated by the Governor, would be the best likely outcome. "The BCMS position is one of support for the concept of binding arbitration as long as the findings of the arbitration panel are admissible in court and carry the presumption of correctness." Several Bills were introduced in 1976, one establishing an arbitration panel that would consider cases in which the claim exceeded $5,000 (but whose decisions were not absolutely binding) and another which would establish a state fund to pay damages up to $100,000, the limit of liability that would be allowed under the law. The former Bill passed, the latter was sent to the Legislative Malpractice Study Committee for summer review.

The year before, Medical Mutual Liability Insurance Society of Maryland was incorporated to "provide relief to the current critical situation by enabling a mutual liability insurance company to be formed...and by establishing an insurance pool to which physicians denied insurance by two companies may apply." Med Mutual was to be the insurer of last resort, and every licensed physician in Maryland was assessed $300 to cover start-up costs. The first policies were mailed May 31, 1975. It was not long, however, before it was recognized that even Med Mutual could not survive under the pressure from plaintiffs, and in spite of the new company, it was still necessary to find a way to rein in awards. The September, 1985 Newsletter notes the "high and rapidly rising professional liability insurance rates."

A total of 6 Bills was introduced in 1986 addressing tort reform. They would establish a mechanism for determining a suit's merit before proceeding to court, limit non-economic awards to $250,000, eliminate punitive damages and adjust the statute of limitations. Ultimately, a $350,000 cap was agreed upon and procedures that would allow structured settlements were put into place. "We hope that this first positive step in meaningful tort reform will encourage the reinsurance carriers to stay in the Maryland marketplace...relieving some upward pressure on premiums," Society President Gary Rosenberg was pleased to announce in April, 1986. Several years earlier, the Society began the practice of providing physicians on a volunteer basis to man the legislative first aid station in Annapolis during the session, reasoning that this presented an ideal opportunity for physicians to act as one-on-one lobbyists with Delegates and Senators.

The next session found Legislative Committee Chairman Dr. Thomas Hunt again encouraging members to write to their legislators. An insurance market basket of Bills was introduced in 1986 that would, if passed, reduce the statute of limitations for minors regarding malpractice suits, allocate the costs associated with arbitration and further define the limit on non-economic damages. The opposition, plaintiff lawyers, had a Bill that would raise the cap that the legislature had set the previous year. The statute of limitations Bill passed, and the cap remain unchanged.

Little by little, the Society's advocates, working alongside the MedChi Legislative Committee and their colleagues from the other components, chipped away at the remaining issues surrounding malpractice insurance and tort reform. The evidentiary standards by which a claim was to be proven was changed from "a preponderance of evidence," to "a standard of clear and convincing." The rates charged by Medical Mutual Liability were adjusted to reflect multiple risk factors rather than being a single rate for every physician, regardless of specialty or history.

The next challenge came in 1994, when the $350,000 cap on non-economic awards was questioned. The cap was to apply to cases of "personal injury," and in a 1993 case the Maryland Court of Appeals ruled that personal injury does not include death. Before that decision, Medical Mutual had found it necessary to file only one rate increase, and had returned $60 million in dividends to its insureds (the covered physicians being the owners of this mutual company). Three Bills were introduced that would have increased the cap to as much as $750,000, and raise it annually at a rate to equal the cost of living increase. By the end of the 1994 session a cap was in place, but it was $500,000 for non-economic awards, $750,000 if the case involved wrongful death, a Pyrrhic victory at best.

Steadily increasing professional liability insurance premiums was the result, bringing the Society to the 2004 session in Annapolis. By then, the $500,000 cap had advanced to $635,000 and physicians were seeking a rollback to the original $350,000 amount. The size of claims had risen nearly 60% in just 3 years and Medical Mutual Liability found itself paying more than double the settlement dollars in the same period. More than 1,500 doctors clogged the streets of Annapolis on January 21, some with white lab coats over their topcoats on a cold Wednesday.

"Right now, soaring payments in the courts are propelling soaring insurance costs, and those costs are damaging our health care system," Dr. Willarda Edwards said before the crowd in Annapolis. Not only had average premiums risen 28% for the year, most physicians could find coverage only from Medical Mutual. (In 1995, there were 14 companies marketing professional medical liability in Maryland).

Proponents and opponents lined up as the session took shape. Governor Robert Ehrlich expressed sympathy for the physicians and the Maryland Chamber of Commerce called for tort reform that would relieve some of the pressure on premiums. The Maryland Trial Lawyers Association, the segment of the Bar which specializes in filing negligence claims, predictably took up arms against reform, backed by a small coterie of victims. At the close of the 2004 session, no action was taken in either the House of Delegates or the State Senate, assuring that tort reform and limits to medical malpractice awards would be on upcoming legislative agendas.

"Physicians as a group are not politically astute. For decades, they have been solely concerned with the daily challenges of providing care to patients as technology and diseases change...Though today's rally may be viewed as naive by some, meager by others, even unprofessional by a few, those of us present will share a common conviction that the health care of all the citizens of Maryland warrants this effort."

-Scott E. Maizel, President
Maryland Chapter of the American College of Surgeons
Commenting on a January 21, 2004 rally
of Maryland physicians calling for tort reform

"Another flagrant disregard of our code refers to Article I, Section 8, which treats the patents and secret nostrums. We are aware that a number of our members, either secretly or openly are engaged in the manufacture and sale to druggists of certain medicines manufactured from private formulas, described as cures or <u>antis</u>. Others have a private understanding with some one druggist regarding the prescribing of some one formula or some pharmacopeia preparation by a name known only to the prescriber and the druggist in question. This compels the patient to patronize this particular druggist or compels other druggists to buy of him this preparation at an advanced price.

This is but another instance of commercialism, which lowers the standing of the profession and helps to rob us of the respect of the community."

-Baltimore City Medical Society Minutes
April 7, 1908

"The holding of shares of stock in a company making and dealing in patented or secret medicines, or the using of their products when prescribing, by which means ultimately receiving a share in the profits of said company, is therefor incompatible with membership in the Baltimore City Medical Society."

-Baltimore City Medical Society
By-Laws, as amended April, 1908

Nostrums and Drugs, Legal and Otherwise

If there is an era in American history that may be called the heyday of patent medicines, miracle cures, soothing syrups, and curative tonics it would surely be the last half of the nineteenth century. A combination of social phenomena conspired to foist upon the American public a vast array of cure-alls which would for a small price relieve the sufferer of everything from asthma to "women's weakness." The post-Civil War economy was strong. The art of lithography was advancing, unfortunately, faster than the science of medicine.

Color advertisements featuring the whiskered assurances of grandfatherly "doctors" and portraits of women engaged in all manner of sports (having overcome "those distressing weaknesses so common to womankind") were more graphically enticing than the remedies offered by legitimate physicians. Truth be told, medicine was still clueless regarding many of the most common, and deadliest, diseases. An understanding of the germ theory of disease was yet cutting edge science, and penicillin was several generations away. "Dr. C. McLane's Celebrated Liver Pills and Vermifuge" probably looked like an attractive alternative to an expensive visit to the surgery.

This was also the era in which the physicians of Baltimore were gathering to form the professional organizations which eventually merged to become the Baltimore City Medical Society. By 1866, when the Baltimore Medical Association was formed, the existence of the American Medical Association, the progress of medicine engendered by the recent Civil War and the advances in education had moved medicine from guesswork to science. Yet the constant battle against snake oil purveyors continued unabated - intensified, in fact. It must have been exasperating for legitimate practitioners to open the *Baltimore American & Commercial Daily Advertiser* and see its pages filled with promises to end diseases that doctors were powerless to cure, and to know that the seemingly-benevolent liars who ran the companies were getting rich in the bargain. The earliest mention in the Association's Minutes of patent medicines came in November, 1872, when a committee was appointed, in partnership with the Medical and Surgical Society of Baltimore, to study the proper relationship between druggists and physicians. Sadly, no record of that committee's proceedings survives.

Government turned a blind eye to the outrageous claims made by patent drug companies, as this was also the period before federal drug regulation. Prior to the Harrison Act of 1914, which was Washington's first foray into the complex arena of drug addiction and abuse, makers of patent medicines were free to spike their secret recipes with morphine, opium, cannabis, cocaine and heroin. If the drug did absolutely nothing to effect a cure, at least the user believed that it was doing something, and that something usually felt good. The first task of organizations like the Baltimore City Medical Society was to alert the public to the false claims of the makers of patent, or proprietary, medications, and to lobby government at every level to force their makers to reveal the contents. The Pure Food and Drug Act of 1906 was a step in the right direction.

Before 1906 there was no regulation whatsoever on the claims manufacturers of over-the-counter products could make. Advertisements featured pictures of well-known people (an ad featuring President Grover Cleveland and his young wife showed Mrs. Cleveland wearing a brooch announcing "Harter's Iron Tonic," re-touched into place according to a printing historian). Many of the medicines that were sold still occupy shelf space in modern pharmacies: Cuticura Ointment, Bromo-Seltzer, Campho-Phenique and Ex-Lax for example. On the eve of the Pure Food and Drug Act's passage, there were an estimated 50,000 patent medicines in use, with a market value in 1998 dollars of $1.4 billion.

The original Pure Food and Drug Act required that certain ingredients, usually the most addictive or potentially toxic, be listed. It fell short in requiring that the government prove inefficacy before a product could be removed from the market. So "Moffat's Vegetable Life Pills" could claim to cure tuberculosis and unless the government could prove in court otherwise, it stayed in the pharmacy.

It took until the 1911 Sherley Amendment, which expressly prohibited making false therapeutic claims to defraud the public, to seal this loophole. Between the original 1906 passage and this amendment, the number of companies manufacturing patent medicines in the United States *increased*, but after a company's ability to make unsubstantiated claims was curtailed, that number plummeted. At the time of the Sherley Amendment, there were approximately 3,000 proprietary medicine companies in business, up by a couple hundred since 1906, and by more than ten-fold since 1870. When the next important amendment passed, the 1938 Food, Drug and Cosmetic Act, the companies had dwindled to under 2,000. As regulations tightened the number dropped further until by 1980, before the merger madness of the 1990's, it had settled at just under a thousand.

As Congress was debating the passage of the Pure Food and Drug Act in 1906, the Baltimore City Medical Society made its first major foray into politics when it lobbied for the passage of a statewide requirement for patent medicine labeling. The effort proved unsuccessful, as the Society was unable to match the political might of Captain Isaac E. Emerson, the maker of Bromo-Seltzer, and his cohorts, but the cudgel was taken up in Washington and within months of the Society's return from Annapolis to Baltimore the Pure Food and Drug Act was enacted.

Congress again addressed the issue of drugs in 1914, this time in an effort to control the use of potentially-addictive narcotics. The February 19, 1915 meeting of the Baltimore City Medical Society was devoted entirely to a review of the "new Federal Anti-Narcotic Law." Mr. James Dennis, legal counsel for the Medical and Chirurgical Faculty, delivered an address entitled "An Explanation of the Law as it Concerns Physicians," which was followed by a talk about the Bill from the pharmacist's viewpoint by Dr. Henry P. Hynson, a prominent Baltimore pharmacist. Judging from the list of members who participated, it was robustly discussed.

The Harrison Act limited the access of the general public to nature's most effective painkillers - opiates such as heroin and morphine. It permitted practitioners to prescribe either drug in "good faith," as long as it was for "legitimate practice." But there was immediate dispute. The Internal Revenue Bureau, which enforced the Harrison Act, decided that maintaining the comfort of existing addicts by prescribing opiates was not "legitimate." Physicians disagreed, but in a series of court actions they failed to keep their privilege of prescribing opiates without great caution, for fear of ending up behind bars. Their plea was, of course, no different than the current practice of methadone maintenance in the United States, and heroin-weaning programs in Europe.

Dr. A.G. Freedom was expelled from the Society in 1908 after having been "indicted, convicted and fined for the illegal sale of cocaine." The Board of Censors examined the records of the States Attorney, and moved that the doctor's Society membership be revoked. It was, though there was no discussion of the beneficial medical applications of cocaine. Three years had passed since the Coca Cola Company de-cocainized their signature product, but cocaine remained in use as a legally prescribed drug, though heavily regulated until 1914.

By 1925 the Society had established a Narcotics Committee, whose principal role it appears was lobbying for changes in the Harrison Act that barred or severely restricted the use of clinically beneficial products. That year, the Committee Chairman, Dr. A.M. Shipley, conducted "an exhaustive study of the literature American and Foreign, together with the inquiry of many physicians, druggists, and drug manufacturers, institutions for the treatment of drug addiction and special writers on this subject," which "led us to the unanimous opinion that Codeine is not a habit forming drug and should be removed from the restrictions imposed in the Harrison Act." An opiate of value as a cough suppressant, codeine was restricted to the same extent as heroin by the Harrison Act. The Society crafted a Resolution approving the report of Dr. Shipley, which was forwarded to the state Faculty, eventually leading to a Resolution introduced at the next Annual Meeting of the AMA.

Heroin, another member of the opiate family, was widely used as a cough suppressant throughout the 1800's. The Harrison Act made it illegal to distribute heroin, declaring that it was of no medical value whatsoever. But in 1927 it became a topic of conversation when the Society received a letter from Dr. Gustave M. Fritz:

> "I am inclosing a letter that I sent to the AMA. Don't you think that in all fairness to ourselves and our patients, we should have Heroin brought back on the market? If you agree with me on this, can't we have a motion passed to authorize sending a letter to the AMA to this effect?"

Dr. Fritz's letter to the national organization is pasted into the Society's Minutes book. "In my opinion, as well as that of hundreds of other doctors, it [heroin] cannot be surpassed and cannot be equaled as a cough sedative." He referred to the 1927 influenza epidemic, reporting that not only had codeine failed to bring relief to his patients, it resulted in the added indignity of giving them constipation in addition to the cough. But heroin, "when obtainable," was very effective.

"It is an outrage...to let some fanatics dictate to us what to prescribe. It is the lack of courage and backbone on the part of the medical fraternity and an unfairness to our patients to sit back and prescribe inferior remedies," wrote Dr. Fritz. Rather than vote in support of a letter to the same effect from the city Society, the members present voted to pass the matter on to the state Faculty for consideration.

America's other drug of choice - alcohol - was outlawed with the passage of the Volstead Act in 1919. The nation was thrown into the Prohibition Years and organized crime reaped the profits. Nationally, the AMA supported the Act, and participated in the rooting out of physicians who prescribed alcohol for "therapeutic purposes," knowing that the eventual use was simply as a recreational beverage (The national organization estimated that only 10% of the prescriptions written between 1919 and repeal in 1933 were for legitimate medical purposes).

The issue of alcohol abuse was not new for the Baltimore City Medical Society. In 1911 a committee was formed to study the problem. The Committee pointed out that treatment was totally inadequate, and that some local physicians had opened facilities for drying out alcoholics that were ineffective and bordered on the unethical. The notion of a "farm" for alcoholics, to be built and operated by the city government, was introduced. In the end, the committee disbanded after referring its recommendations to the Medical and Chirurgical Faculty.

As lobbying for a national act to ban the sale of alcohol grew, members of both the Baltimore City Medical Society and the Baltimore County Medical Society traveled to Washington for a joint meeting with their District of Columbia colleagues. At the Raleigh Hotel, in May, 1917, a motion was made by Dr. J.H. Drach, a member of the County society, to "ask that the combined societies put themselves on record as in favor of the discontinuance of the manufacture of all alcoholic liquors." No vote was taken, and a decision instead was made to refer it to the various Executive Committees. "Owing to the lateness of the hour," the last scientific report of the evening was canceled. Throughout the 13 years that Prohibition was in effect, the mention of alcoholic beverages was not included in any of the Society's Minutes.

But another popular recreational drug did come under the purview of the Baltimore City Medical Society six years after America reopened the saloon doors. By 1937, the public had been aroused to the dangers of marijuana in a campaign that was part science, part racism, part classism, but mostly fear. When the film *Reefer Madness* was screened in 1938 a face, albeit hugely melodramatic, was attached to the "scourge."

Marijuana had been declared illegal by the 1937 Marijuana Tax Act. "There are 100,000 total marijuana smokers in the United States, and most are Negroes, Hispanics, Philipinos and entertainers. Their Satanic music, jazz and swing, result from marijuana use," the Commissioner of Narcotics testified before Congress in August, 1937. The issue was too important to be ignored by physicians. Cannabis, though not in cigarette form, was widely prescribed for a variety of medicinal purposes prior to 1937.

The American Medical Association went on record in opposition to the Bill that would criminalize marijuana possession without an appropriate tax stamp. In a July, 1937 letter to United States Senator Pat Hoffman, Chairman of the Committee of Finance, in which medical legislation was crafted, the Association's legal counsel laid out the protest:

> "I have been instructed by the Board of Trustees of the American Medical Association to protest on behalf of the association against the enactment in its present form of so much of H.R. 6906 as relates to the medicinal use of cannabis and its preparations and derivatives. The act is entitled 'An Act to impose an occupational excise tax upon certain dealers in marihuana, to impose a transfer tax upon certain dealings in marihuana, and to safeguard the revenue therefrom by registry and recording.'"

The letter continued, claiming that there was no credible evidence that cannabis was addictive, and that the imposition of another layer of paperwork and taxation had the obvious purpose of ending its use altogether. "Since the medicinal use of cannabis has not caused and is not causing addiction, the prevention of the use of the drug for medicinal purposes can accomplish no good end whatsoever. How far it may serve to deprive the public of the benefits of a drug that on further research may prove to be of substantial value, it is impossible to foresee," it concluded.

"The motion picture you are about to witness may startle you. It would not have been possible, otherwise, to sufficiently emphasize the frightful toll of the new drug menace which is destroying the youth of America in alarmingly-increasing numbers. Marihuana is

that drug - a violent narcotic - an unspeakable scourge - The Real Public Enemy Number One!

Its first effect is sudden, violent, uncontrollable laughter; Then come dangerous hallucinations - space expands - time slows down, almost stands still...Fixed ideas come next, conjuring up monstrous extravagances - followed by emotional disturbances, the total inability to direct thoughts, the loss of all power to resist physical emotions...Leading finally to acts of shocking violence....Ending often in incurable insanity. In picturing its soul-destroying effects no attempt was made to equivocate. The scenes are incidents, while fictionalized for the purposes of this story, are based upon actual research into the results of Marihuana addiction. If their stark reality will make you think, will make you aware that something must be done to wipe out this ghastly menace, then the picture will not have failed in its purpose. Because the dread Marihuana may be reaching forth next for your son and daughter."
          -from the introductory screen of the film *Reefer Madness*
          Federal Bureau of Narcotics, 1937

The Baltimore City Medical Society did not formally address the issue of marijuana use until two years after the passage of the Marijuana Tax Act in 1937. But the drug, after having been ignored for years, was in the press on a regular basis beginning in about 1935 and physicians in Baltimore could not possibly have been ignorant of the public furor over it.

Until 1937 it was perfectly legal to use marijuana. The initial publicity about its alleged danger came straight from the office of Harry Anslinger, the Director of the Federal Bureau of Narcotics from its creation in 1930 until 1962. One theory is that its purpose was to increase the Bureau's budget and political clout, a theory supported by the Bureau's obvious use of racial propaganda (the suggestion was made that marijuana only became a threat when white kids took up the habit) to whip up public fury.

Reefer Madness, a "drug education" film, was released by the Bureau in 1937. It depicts a group of religious, upright white high school students who become swept up in the marijuana craze, urged on by a couple of shady operators who maintain a party apartment and sell the drug. Wildly theatrical, in the style of earlier silent cinema, it tells the story of one young man in particular who after just several puffs goes insane and commits murder. The film received wide distribution, but its real impact came thirty years later. Revived as a cult classic, *Reefer Madness* then served to convince the pot smokers of the flower-power generation that the government had no idea about marijuana.

A "Symposium on Marihuana" occupied the scientific agenda of the Society on February 3, 1939. Guest speakers included the Honorable Rowland K. Adams, Judge of the Supreme Bench of Baltimore, Manfred S. Guttmacher, the Supreme Bench's Chief Medical Officer and H.J. Wollner, a Consulting Chemist from the Bureau of Narcotics. The Minutes record only that the Symposium occurred, saying nothing about its content. Apparently, the Society chose not to craft a Resolution pro or con. The law was already in effect, the AMA's lobbying notwithstanding, and doctors had to learn the procedures for the continued medicinal prescribing of the drug. After the Society's symposium there is no further mention of marijuana in its proceedings.

There is, in fact, little mention of the abuse of addictive drugs at all until 1969. Dr. George Vash, wrote a Resolution that year recognizing the epidemic use of heroin on city streets. The population he described could have been found any day on the sidewalk outside his South Gilmor Street surgery: "...unstable, father-deprived families...poorly educated and motivated 'drop-outs' who have not learned how to work and how to play...social, neurotic and psychotic addicts."

What Dr. Vash proposed was a revolutionary concept in the treatment of drug addiction. Methadone was being prescribed by physicians, but treated no differently than morphine, "fraught with the same injunctions." Dr. Vash called for a reform of the current treatment methods, which consisted chiefly of incarceration in an institution where the availability of drugs was probably nearly as widespread as on the streets of southwest Baltimore. While there were some successes, Dr.Vash believed that "the cutting off of family, work and personal ties results in the rapid resumption of the habit after discharge from the resented confinement."

He advocated instead the treatment of addicts by private physicians, supplemented by lay groups in a support capacity, and urged the Baltimore City Medical Society to endorse the establishment of a registry of narcotics offenders, make narcotics addiction a reportable disease rather than a crime, enlist the assistance of the State Laboratory in conducting urinalyses, assign epidemiologists to cases to help primary care givers with follow-up, and create a lawful authority under which physicians be permitted to freely prescribe methadone replacement therapy.

Dr. Vash was perhaps ahead of his time. The Baltimore City Medical Society, rather than approve his resolution, accepted the explanation of Dr. Louis Kolodner, Chair of the state Faculty Committee on Narcotic Prescribing Practices, that the Faculty was adequately addressing the issue. A decision to send the Resolution back to Dr. Vash so that it could be reworded in a fashion acceptable to the Medical and Chirurgical Faculty, was endorsed. Within months, the Society voted to reject the Vash Resolution.

The reprisal from Dr. Vash's South Gilmor Street office was swift and pointed. Federal Narcotics Agents complained that physicians were the source of most of the illegal methadone sold in the black market. They summarily instructed physicians to cease prescribing it, and according to Dr.Vash "Now, that we have stopped prescribing methadone, the black market is as alive as ever, and the harsh 'stop-it-all' order of the Subcommittee has led to frequent relapses to heroin, or flagrant overmedication as practiced by 'ADAPT' and 'MAN ALIVE'." These were two lay organizations in Baltimore that, in spite of documented cases of lax supervision, were allowed to continue distributing methadone. Dr. Vash petulantly withdrew his Resolution.

Over the next four years, however, the Society came to recognize the city's growing problem of narcotics addiction. No doubt the Civil Rights Movement, with the resulting social recognition of African Americans' rights, made it difficult to ignore. In addition, narcotics use was spreading beyond the minority communities of Baltimore. Dr. Vash's office, for instance, was in a mostly Caucasian neighborhood. A Committee on Drugs was created in 1972:

> "There is an immediate need to distinguish 'user' from 'abuser' from 'addict', as well as to discuss drugs and drug categories separately, rather than grouping everything together under drug abuse. There is a vast difference between the adolescent who smokes marijuana once in awhile and the hard core heroin addict and the middle class 'speed freak'."

In 1973 the Committee on Drugs mounted a program geared for health care professionals at North Charles General Hospital which discussed not only the physician's role in treating addiction but also the potential of a physician's being implicated in the creation of the problem ("The Significance of the Prescribing Patterns of Physicians in Problems of Drug Abuse" being one topic). In the late 1960's the Society was notified by federal officials that eight of its members were being investigated for abusive prescription practices, and though there is no record of the outcome of the investigation, the medical community took notice.

Drug issues nearly disappeared through the remainder of the twentieth century. The Society's efforts had been for decades spent exposing the bogus claims of snake oil salesmen, improving relationships between physicians and legitimate druggists, and distinguishing between drugs that offered only recreational utility versus medicinal value. Pure pharmacological science appeared sporadically on the agenda: Organ transplantation obviously demanded an understanding of drugs that could solve the problem of organ rejection. The efficacy of generic drugs as opposed to brand name products became a criteria in determining the Society's support or rejection of insurance legislation. The excesses in prescribing diet drugs was examined.

These topics were covered from a scientific point of view. Presentations on the role of the medical community vis-a-vis substance abuse were medically, rather than morally or legally, oriented. The administrator for substance abuse programs for the city's Department of Health and Human Services delivered an address entitled "Pharmacological Calvinism" in 1980. In 1986, Dr. Raymond F. Contee, Chairman of the Medical Advisory Board for the U.S. Department of Transportation, talked to the membership about "Disease, Drugs, Driving and Doctors."

"Snake Oil," 1980's Style

Harken back to 1906, just before the passage of the Pure Food and Drug Act, when the Baltimore City Medical Society was embroiled in a battle for honesty in advertising, and for printed lists of ingredients on patent medicine containers. Now fast forward 75 years, for that is how long it took for the patent medicine industry to resurface, with outlandish claims of the efficacy of "The Dyna-Slim Fat Liquidation Plan." "An amazing weight loss pill that will enable virtually anyone to reduce easily - without trying to diet, without having to give up favorite foods," the advertisements of the Consumer Publishing Company boasted. The Society took note of the outlandish assertions made for "The Ultimate Diet Pill," and called them to the attention of the Consumer Protection Division of the Maryland Office of the Attorney General.

Hearings were called in Annapolis, and three members of the Society were on hand to testify. Dyna-Slim was, they said, based on evidence just about as "scientific" as that used in 1900 to back up the claim by the Cafeeno Company that their product would cure colon cancer. Shortly thereafter an order was issued calling for the cessation of advertisements by the Consumer Publishing Company, doing business as Weight Loss Center, National Pharamacols and Richelieu Pharmacols, and ending the sale of their weight loss product. The order required that the company "restore to all residents of Maryland who have purchased any products in response to the advertisement...the purchase price, including postage, of such products." "Sometimes," Dr. Henry Wagner proudly reported, "something can be done about it."

In 2004, DynaSlim advertised on the internet as a weight loss patch, by a company in the United Kingdom, not likely to be the original American manufacturer. "Ephedra Free," "All Natural Ingredients" its box proclaimed. When the web surfer clicked on the manufacturer's url, www.dynaslim.com, he or she ended up at a site which advertises that, with their help, anyone can sell anything on the internet. Among the products offered: "Q-Ray Bracelets," "Vigorelle," "Ultra Hair Away." The internet: A new world for purveyors of miracle cures and snake oil.

"The active ingredient in DynaSlim is fucus vesiculosis, a marine algae found off the coasts of England and Ireland...DynaSlim is included in such publications as The Homeopathic Review, Allen's Encyclopedia of Pure Materia Medica, The Pharmacopeia of the American Institute of Homeopathy, and the United States Homeopathic Pharmacopeia."

-from the DynaSlim website, 2004

"...to support the aims of the medical society, in all of its efforts to advance the standards of community health and to promote a closer relationship among the physicians' families which would make for a feeling of local cooperation."

-from the organizational documents of the
Baltimore City Medical Society Woman's Auxiliary

"The Baltimore City Medical Society should form a non-profit corporation which could accept tax deductible contributions. Funds so received would be used for various educational and public health projects."

-from a 1972 BCMS Resolution, unanimously adopted

"The wives of Baltimore doctors, accompanying their husbands to medical meetings and scientific seminars, have for years envied the women of other communities the pleasure which they obviously derived from the auxiliaries to their local medical societies."

-Mrs. George H. Yeager
in an interview for the Evening Sun
March 6, 1950

The Baltimore City Medical Society Auxiliary and the Baltimore City Medical Society Foundation

Forty-seven states had woman's auxiliaries in place in their local components before the Baltimore City Medical Society established its own, on October 9, 1949, with 99 charter members. Even then, the group was begun only at the suggestion of the Medical and Chirurgical Faculty. "Baltimore...true to its reputation for ultra-conservatism, was the last to do anything about it," admitted the Auxiliary's first president, Mrs. George H. Yeager (whose husband, Dr. George H. Yeager, was editor of the *Maryland State Medical Journal*).

As the country, and the city, moved through the prosperity and peace of the 1950's into the tumult of the Vietnam years and beyond, and as the focus of the Baltimore City Medical Society gradually shifted from science and education to advocacy and legislation, several adjunct organizations were formed to address projects which were no longer on the Society's main radar screen. The first was the Woman's Auxiliary (later, just the Auxiliary, still later, the Alliance). It was followed in 1972 by the Baltimore City Medical Society Foundation, as well as the short-lived Management Services Corporation.

The Auxiliary's mission statement described an organization which was to serve in an associate capacity to advance the mission of the Society. Informally, the Auxiliary was to serve another purpose, that being to integrate the wives of physicians newly relocated to Baltimore City or who opened new city practices with the existing social circle of other spouses. "Many young women from out of town who have moved here with doctor husbands, have remarked that, while doctors' wives who are old Baltimoreans may have no actual need to widen their acquaintance, newcomers would appreciate an opportunity to meet the wives of their husband's colleagues in the Baltimore City Medical Society."

Mrs. Yeager and the Auxiliary jumped into their role in support of the Society's mission with both feet, becoming a jack-of-all-trades that handled everything from planning cruises to installing seatbelts to collecting pharmaceutical products to send to missions in Africa. However, there is no mention whatsoever of the Auxiliary in the general Minutes of the Society in its first year The Society By-Laws were never changed to give the Auxiliary any representation on the Society's Board of Directors. An Advisory Council to the Woman's Auxiliary was eventually formed, but in its early years it reported having had no meetings of consequence. It was explicit in the extent of its control, however: "The duties...shall be that of counselor and advisor on all projects of the Woman's Auxiliary and on all matters concerning policy, none of which shall be executed without the approval of this advisory committee."

The first Auxiliary entry in the Society's budget did not appear until 1952, when an expense of $5.00 was recorded with no detailed explanation, offset by the receipt of $5.00 in dues from the Auxiliary. Incoming presidents failed in their annual addresses to recognize the Auxiliary until 1953, when Dr. Wetherbee Fort wrote, "I am also happy to announce that the Woman's Auxiliary to the Baltimore City Medical Society, at their own time, trouble and expense, will serve coffee and doughnuts after all of our meetings next year..." In 1961, when the Auxiliary proposed ballroom dancing lessons in the Faculty headquarters, the Executive Committee thought not. Selling Christmas cards was one thing, waltzes in Osler Hall apparently quite another. Events that were still beneath the perceived dignity of the profession, such as publicity and fundraising, became the role of the Auxiliary.

However, the Society was quick to call upon the Auxiliary when needed, and equally willing to thank their spouses for their service. Dr. Amos Koontz, in 1951, wrote the first of several Resolutions honoring the women's contributions:

> "WHEREAS, the Woman's Auxiliary to the Baltimore City Medical Society have been untiring in their efforts to aid the work of the Society in manifold ways, such as in the fight against socialized medicine and the fight for the preservation of medical research, to mention only two;
>
> BE IT RESOLVED, that the Baltimore City Medical Society wishes to express its heartiest thanks to all the ladies for their great devotion, untiring energy, and invaluable aid..."

To conclude from the sparse recognition of the Auxiliary in the general Minutes, however, that the Auxiliary was not active, would be incorrect. In 1954 there were 17 standing committees, and many of them - including Legislation, Medical Research, Nurse Scholarship, Mental Hygiene and Civil Defense - were far beyond mere refreshments and fashion shows. From the beginning the Auxiliary was determined to participate in the serious aspects of medicine, with a concentration on topics of public health. The quarterly meetings opened with a talk on some public health project (Dr. Dean Roberts addressed an early Auxiliary luncheon on the Maryland Medical Care Program for the Indigent, "which is considered a model for the nation"). Members of the Woman's Auxiliary sponsored events that discussed poliomyelitis (1954), Juvenile Delinquency (1954), "Ronald Reagan Speaks out against Socialized Medicine" (1961) and "Planned Parenthood and the Population Problem" (1968).

An early and important initiative of the Auxiliary came in 1953. At the first Executive Committee meeting of the year, a proposal was discussed that the Society fund a "nurse recruitment film," to be created and distributed by the Auxiliary. The Committee thought enough of the idea to add it to the agenda of the next general meeting, where an allocation of $50.00 toward the project was approved. The result was "The Girl with the Lamp," a color film produced by the Auxiliary in cooperation with the Maryland Society for Medical Research and the technical assistance of the Maryland State Nurses Association.

The film documented the life of a student nurse, following her through her training and presenting the career options for nurses outside the hospital. It was followed up by the establishment of a Nurse Student Aid Fund in 1954. A new print of the film was purchased by the Auxiliary in 1958, and the Society, in agreeing to cover the $150.00 cost, recognized the film's importance.

"WHEREAS, as is their annual custom, the Woman's Auxiliary to the Baltimore City Medical Society will sponsor the observance of the day in recognition of the contributions made by doctors to the Nation's health and well-being..." With this proclamation, Baltimore Mayor Thomas D'Alesandro, Jr. recognized "Doctors' Day in Baltimore," on March 30, 1955. The year closed with a holiday art sale, sponsored by the Auxiliary, and a note that the Auxiliary's cocktail party at the previous Annual Meeting was a "huge success," but perhaps when it was repeated the expense could be reduced "by having a less expensive hors d'oeuvre."

By 1957 the Auxiliary launched the first scholarship program in the Society's long history. The first fundraiser, a benefit concert by the Baltimore Symphony Orchestra, resulted in the establishment of two annual scholarships in the amount of $250 each, one to go to a worthy student at Hopkins and the other to a student at the University of Maryland. A program that extended small loans to medical students, none greater than $1,000, was also started, and books carrying loan balances and showing periodic payments were kept well into the 1990's. The scholarship function of the Auxiliary was eventually supplanted by the creation of the Baltimore City Medical Society Foundation, whose legal structure gave it much greater fundraising capacity.

A multitude of other projects filled the Auxiliary's schedule over the years. There were card parties and fashion shows. Auxiliary members performed the can-can at the MedChi Ball, "An Evening in Paris," in 1952. A one-act play, "Private Lives of Doctor's Wives," was written and performed in 1954. Every year featured a Ball - the Mardi Gras Ball, the Tiara Ball, the Red Slipper Ball. The events made the society pages in all of the local newspapers, none more so than when the Auxiliary mounted an automobile seatbelt campaign in May, 1963. For $3.88, members provided and installed seatbelts on the Memorial Stadium parking lot. Baltimore Orioles third baseman Brooks Robinson was shown in the *Sun*, snapping his seatbelt closed for the first time.

When MedChi changed the name of its spouse's group from Auxiliary to Alliance, the Baltimore City Medical Society did the same. By that time, membership and Alliance programs were on the wane, and the scholarship program had moved to the agenda of the Foundation. The Alliance's last official responsibility was raising funds to contribute to the scholarship pool, but by 1999 interest was so minimal that the Alliance disbanded.

The Baltimore City Medical Society Foundation is Born

Scholarships proved to be the permanent legacy of the Woman's Auxiliary, continuing unabated within the general structure of the Baltimore City Medical Society until the Baltimore City Medical Society Foundation was formed in 1972. The amounts grew to $1,000 in 1972, when a Hopkins-bound student was chosen by a committee of the Baltimore City Public Schools. The need to raise funds for scholarships made necessary the creation of a 501(c)(3) non-profit legal entity that could accept tax-deductible donations for the purpose, and in September, 1974 the first call went out for contributions to get the Foundation started. "The BCMS Foundation is a philanthropic organization formed to support scholarships, special post-graduate educational activities, public health programs and other worthwhile medically-oriented projects," the call for donations explained.

By 1975 there were sufficient funds to begin a search for the

Foundation's first scholarship recipients. A letter went out to financial aid offices at medical schools across the country. Prospective recipients needed a permanent Baltimore City address, and had to be enrolled in an accredited medical or osteopathy school. The first two recipients, a student at Howard University and another at Johns Hopkins, received grants totaling $1,500 in 1976. As the fund grew so did the awards. In 1977, five students shared a total of $4,000, and in 1981 scholarships spread among four students reached $5,000. Eight students benefitted from the Foundation's programs in 1990, when a total of $12,000 was granted.

The Foundation also sought out worthy non-scholarship programs. They were nominal at first, but grew as the Foundation's resources increased. The first grant, $100 to the Baltimore City Alliance Against Venereal Diseases in 1973, financed that group's Baltimore City Fair booth. In 1989 the Foundation donated $1000 to Health Care for the Homeless. Three groups received Foundation funds in 1994, sharing $7,250. That year the Foundation reported an especially successful fundraising campaign and "increased contributions by individual members, their friends and families, and by hospital medical staffs and several specialty societies."

When the Homewood Hospitals closed in 1991, the balance in the institutions' charitable accounts was donated to the Baltimore City Medical Society Foundation to support an annual scholarship. In June, Dr. Ruth Ashman, the last President of the Homewood Hospital staff, presented the Foundation with a check for $75,000. The medical staffs at North Charles General Hospital and the Wyman Park Medical Associates, the institutions which made up Homewood Hospitals, had voted to donate all of the funds left in its treasury after the medical center's final expenses were paid. Dr. Beryl Rosenstein, the President of the BCMS Foundation at the time, along with Dr. Philip Wagley, who chaired the committee which created the Foundation in 1972, accepted the check.

Other significant contributions enabled the Foundation to bolster its yearly giving. Three scholarships were funded annually by gifts in memory of three Baltimore physicians who were long time city practitioners: Drs. Elliot R. Fishel (President of the Society in 1985), Nathan E. Needle, and Kennard L. Yaffe (Society President in 1983). A strategic plan was set up during the Foundation Presidency of Dr. Murray Kalish (1993-1996) to solicit donations from hospital medical staffs, and every hospital in Baltimore participated. Allied specialty societies were contacted, with Dr. Kalish's own Maryland-District of Columbia Society of Anesthesiologists making the first $1,000 specialty society donation. The Foundation then turned to local corporations for donations.

The much-appreciated boosts in the Foundation's assets allowed a gradual increase in the generosity of the scholarships: 1993, $15,750, increasing to $42,000 in 1995. By 1999, the total scholarships granted by the Foundation since its inception reached $212,000, having provided assistance for 53 students.

"When I was notified that I was awarded the scholarship, I was ecstatic."

-Mary I. Jumbelic, M.D.
From a February, 2004 letter

It is hard to know where to begin my story but I will make a stab at it. Thank you for allowing me this opportunity to express my gratitude to the society for their generosity during my medical training.

I was born, raised, and lived in Baltimore for 29 years. Since I was 13 years old, I carried the dream of becoming a doctor. My father died that year and I often visited him at the hospital, where I would observe the men in white taking care of him. He had chronic heart and lung disease, having been a coal miner and then a house painter for most of his life. He only completed the 8th grade and my mother graduated high school, so they encouraged me to go farther with my education than they were able.

The years of college and medical school were very difficult financially for my mother and me. She worked as a maid and then as a keypunch operator at near minimum wage.

I worked part time jobs since the age of 13, first selling flowers at a corner stall, helping my mother clean doctors' offices on weekends, and even as an answering service operator throughout high school servicing many Baltimore doctors.

I lived at home to save the cost of campus housing and traveled daily to the University of Maryland, Baltimore County, a 45 minute trip each way from Northeast Baltimore. My mother changed jobs so she could take public transportation, and I could have the family car. I held part time jobs throughout college to help defray the cost of tuition and our living expenses. Medical school was an even more difficult burden, and I took out loans to be able to attend, still living at home the first semester to save money.

I remember applying for the Baltimore City Medical Society Scholarship and feeling nervous about the outcome. It literally made the difference between needing a part time job or focusing my energies on my education. When I was notified that I was awarded the scholarship, I was ecstatic. My mother and I attended a dinner reception to honor the awardees. I felt awkward, coming from a blue collar background into a world of what I perceived to be high society. Yet the sincerity and generosity with which the award was given alleviated my concerns. The scholarship was essential to providing necessary funding for my medical school education.

Now, 20 years after my graduation from medical school, as the Chief Medical Examiner in Syracuse, New York, I remember with gratitude the BCMS and the money that was so generously provided to me to help me through medical school. It was given to me simply because my family needed it. I hold my medical degree in high honor and am proud to carry the title of doctor. *The scholarship truly helped fulfill my lifelong dream.*

Dr. Mary I. Jumbelic was the recipient of scholarship assistance from the Baltimore City Medical Society Foundation for four years beginning in 1979.

As the Foundation's philanthropy grew it broadened its fundraising agenda even further. The first BCMS Foundation Golf Tournament was held on June 21, 2000 at Baltimore's Mount Pleasant Golf Course. The tournament, which has since become an annual event, was supported by 27 sponsors including pharmaceutical companies, hospitals, managed care companies and local financial institutions. Dr. Reed Winston, President of the Society the following year, chaired the first tournament and captained the third place men's team. Dr. Eve Higginbotham, who presided over the Society in 2003, led the winning women's foursome (Dr. Higginbotham also won closest to the pin).

In addition to its scholarships, the Foundation began publishing the Society's public medical education newsletter in 1988. Launched as *Info Med, Health Information Service of the Baltimore City Medical Society*, the quarterly newsletter featured articles written by BCMS members and others on a broad range of personal health topics, as well as columns to help patients find their way through the ever-increasing maze of health insurance providers, HMOs, PPOs, and all the other acronyms of modern medicine. The premier issue featured an article by Dr. John Meyerhoff reminding readers that the season for flu shots had arrived. BCMS Executive Director Bernadette Huber Lane contributed a short column explaining how Medicare set physician fees, and how that schedule impacted the amounts that physicians charged non-Medicare patients. Newsletters were purchased by physicians to provide their patients with accurate, easy-to-understand information that would help them become better health care consumers.

The logo was updated and the name changed to *BCMS Report* in the summer of 1991. The content, however, remained the same. Society officers received frequent bylines, Dr. Donald Dembo in 1992 for "Tools To Test Your Heart," Dr. Beverly Collins in 1999 for "Beware of 'Natural' Weight-loss Products." Dr. Meyerhoff dusted off his flu shot reminder occasionally as the season and the threat demanded. The Foundation, working with the Action for Community Enrichment Coalition, established centers across Baltimore where citizens could receive flu shots at no charge. The majority of the articles were, and continue to be, the work of physicians who do not serve in leadership positions with the Society. The result is a selection of topics wider in scope than might otherwise have been possible, including not only articles about recent developments in curative medicine but also many pieces about preventive medicine as well.

In 1998, at the suggestion of the chairperson of the Society's Public Information Committee, Dr. Henry Meilman, the Foundation funded an ambitious program to train Baltimore City high school students in cardiopulmonary resuscitation. In partnership with the Baltimore City Fire Academy, over 500 students whose majors were in health care received CPR training in the first four years of the program.

The BCMS Foundation marked its 33rd year of benevolent giving as the Society celebrated its centennial in 2004. At the close of 2003, 76 medical students had received a total of $259,500 over that 33-year period from the BCMS Foundation.

"As I mentioned earlier, medical and nursing school scholarships are one of our ongoing programs. We continue to publish our patient newsletter, BCMS Report. *It is distributed through our offices, as well as public health clinics, senior citizen residences, eating together programs and the Pratt Library System. We also provide CPR instruction in the City high schools and work with the American Heart Association on Operation Heartbeat to increase the number of individuals trained in CPR. With the Bar Association, we visit elementary and middle schools to talk with students about the dangers of drugs. We are looking to build on these programs as we begin our 32nd year in 2004..."*

    -Dr. Marshall Bedine, President of the BCMS Foundation
    speaking at the BCMS Annual Meeting, November, 2003

"...The days when people in academic medicine could remain in their ivory towers in splendid isolation from the world about them are gone forever. All of us - practicing, public health and academic physicians - must now join forces if we are to continue our progress toward better health care, better education, and better research."

-Dr. Henry N. Wagner
President's Viewpoint, January, 1980

PRESIDENTS OF BALTIMORE MEDICAL SOCIETIES

Before 1866 (Dates of service are difficult to document for pre-1866 medical societies):

Charles Frederick (Friedrich) Wiesenthal, M.D. (1726-1789)
Family history reported that Dr. Wiesenthal was Surgeon to Frederick the Great before emigrating to Baltimore from his native Germany in 1755. Upon his arrival, he immediately became a public figure within and without the small medical community. He served on the Baltimore Committee of Correspondence and was Surgeon-General to the Maryland troops throughout the American Revolution. In 1779, at the height of the American Revolution, Dr. Weisenthal mounted a campaign to apprize the public of the difficulties imposed on the profession by the war, and organized the first "Red Cross," in which citizens rolled bandages and assisted with wounded troops. In the late 1780's, he created the first, albeit short-lived, Baltimore medical society. From his Fayette Street residence, Dr. Wiesenthal conducted the first "medical school" in the city, which was continued after his death by his son. He has often been called "The Father of the Medical Profession in Baltimore."

Andrew Wiesenthal, M.D. (1762-1798)
The younger Dr. Wiesenthal, who was born in Baltimore, attended lectures in Philadelphia and Great Britain before returning to Baltimore to take over his father's apprenticeship-based anatomy school. He and his partner, Dr. George Buchanan, are credited with preserving the European type of medical teaching which would eventually form the foundation of the curriculum at the University of Maryland.

Dr. George Augustus Dunkel (17? - 1838)
A native of Westphalia, Germany, Dr. Dunkle was, with Dr. John

Beale Davidge, one of the founders of the 1804 Medical Society of Baltimore.

William Donaldson, M.D. (1778-1835)
Dr. Donaldson graduated from St. John's College in Annapolis in 1798, studied in Baltimore under Dr. Miles Littlejohn and attended lectures at the University of Pennsylvania. One of the Founders of the College of Medicine in Maryland, he also served as President of the Medical Society of Baltimore from 1822-1823.

Samuel Baker, M.D. (1785-1835)
Samuel Baker, M.D. was a Baltimore native who studied under Drs. Littlejohn and Donaldson (see above). He studied at Washington College in Chestertown, Maryland and the University of Pennsylvania. Dr. Baker was on the first faculty at the University of Maryland and its precursor, the Maryland Medical College, until 1830, President of the Baltimore Medical Society and Secretary of the Medical and Chirurgical Faculty of Maryland. He is credited with having created the Faculty's first library.

John Lloyd Yeates, M.D. (1802-1875)
Receiving his medical degree from the University of Maryland in 1822, Dr. Yeates was not only a member of the Baltimore City Council but President of the state Medical and Chirurgical Faculty from 1853-1854. He presided over the Medical and Surgical Society of Baltimore from 1855 - 1856. Dr. Yeates' obituary reported that in 1860 "He experienced a severe attack of paralysis from which he never fully recovered, though he was still able, for some years, to render service and advice to old friends and patients."

"The Late Distinguished Ornament and Acknowledged Head of our Profession"

NATHAN RYNO SMITH, M.D. (1797-1877)

While never having presided over a local Baltimore medical society, Dr. Nathan Ryno Smith figured prominently in the careers of many other distinguished Baltimore physicians. His name was one that appeared in other practitioners' obituaries more frequently than in his own: "A student of Dr. Nathan Ryno Smith," a single phrase which was enough to advise the reader that the deceased was a doctor of distinction and high professional achievement.

Born in Cornish, New Hampshire, Dr. Smith took his baccalaureate degree at Yale and received his medical degree from the same institution in 1823. Just two years later he founded the Medical Department at the University of Vermont in Burlington, where he had set up his practice. In 1827 he began a 50-year affiliation with the University of Maryland, as Professor of Surgery, President of the Faculty and Dean. Dr. Smith was President of the Medical and Chirurgical Faculty from 1870-1872, and during his long career he edited both the *Philadelphia Journal of Medicine and Surgery* and that journal's counterpart in Baltimore.

One of his students, Samuel Claggett Chew, M.D., in an address to the state Faculty in 1878, recalled his mentor fondly. "You can recall Professor Smith as he appeared so often on consultation...that rare diagnostic skill with which he steered his conclusions almost by intuition. In your mind's eye you can see him discoursing in the ampitheatre in the attitude of dignity and command which always belonged to him. He has left behind him the record of a great surgeon, a brave and true citizen, a magnanimous gentleman."

Baltimore Medical Association (The year in which the physician was Association President appears before the name):

1866 - Gerald Edwin Morgan, M.D. (1828-1874)
Shortly after his 1852 graduation from Washington Medical College, Dr. Morgan became a vaccine physician in Baltimore. He served as Assistant Health Commissioner of Baltimore from 1861-1862, then moved to the Commissioner's office from 1865-1867. "The poor were especially his friends," an 1879 biographer wrote, confirmed by his volunteer work as surgeon at The Boy's Home, and "one of the originators of summer excursions for the poor." Dr. Morgan was a Founder and the first President of the Baltimore Medical Association. He was Vice President of the Medical and Chirurgical Faculty at the time of his death in 1874. The Baltimore Medical Association drafted a Resolution at its December 14 meeting that year in his honor: "This Association has been deprived of an honourable and useful member, the community has lost a good citizen, and the poor a generous and ever-ready friend."

1867 - Philip C. Williams, M.D. (1828-1896)
Educated at the University of Maryland and the University of Pennsylvania, Dr. Williams was an early President of the Baltimore Medical Association and a Founder of the Baltimore Clinical Society (1873). He presided over the Medical and Chirurgical Faculty from 1872-1873, after which he became President of the Baltimore Pathological Society.

1868 - Andrew Hartman, M.D. (1816-1884)
After receiving his baccalaureate from Pennsylvania College in Gettysburg, Dr. Hartman continued his studies at the Washington Medical College in Baltimore. He served as Vice President of the Medical and Chirurgical Faculty from 1872-1873.

1869 - Charles Hyland Jones, M.D. (1828-1897)
Dr. Charles Hyland Jones came to Baltimore from Somerset County, on the lower Maryland Eastern Shore, to study at the Baltimore Medical Institute and the University of Maryland. A Founder of the Baltimore Medical Association, he also served three terms as Vice President of the state Faculty.

1870 - James Hamilton Curry (Currey), M.D. (1832-1887)
Another of the Founders of the Baltimore Medical Association in 1866, Dr. Curry came to Baltimore from Frederick, Maryland. He was granted his M.D. degree from the University of Maryland in 1859. He was President of the Baltimore City Medical Association and served often as a state delegate to the American Medical Association

1871 - Abraham (Abram) B. Arnold, M.D. (1820-1904)
Arriving in Baltimore from Wurttemberg, Germany in 1832, Dr. Arnold attended lectures at both the University of Pennsylvania and the Washington University of Medicine, where he earned his medical degree in 1848. He assumed the Vice Presidency of the state Faculty in 1872, finally rising to the Faculty's Presidency in 1877. "A writer of much force and ability," Dr. Arnold's byline appeared often in medical journals, on topics including "Cholera Infantum," and "Poisoning by Cyanide of Potassium." Dr. Arnold authored *The Manual of Nervous Diseases*, written while he was a consulting physician at Hebrew Hospital.

1872 - Thomas Sargent Latimer, M.D. (1839-1906)
Born in Savannah, Georgia, Dr. Latimer served in the Confederate States of America Army during the Civil War. After the war he returned to Baltimore, where he had received his medical degree in 1861, and began a long academic career on the faculties of the Baltimore College of Dental Surgery, the College of Physicians and Surgeons and Baltimore Polyclinic. As a surgeon, he filled staff positions at the Nursery and Child's Hospital and the Baltimore Infirmary. From 1872-1873 he was President of the Baltimore Medical Association, was Vice President of the state Faculty from 1882-1883 and the following year served as the Faculty's President. Dr. Latimer edited the *Baltimore Medical Journal* and *Physician and Surgeon*.

1873 - John Reese Uhler, M.D. (1839-?)
Receiving his medical degree from the University of Maryland in 1861, just in time to begin a 4-year enlistment in the Union Army, Dr. Uhler returned to post-war Baltimore to teach at Baltimore Medical College and to assume the Superintendent's position at

Bayview Asylum. From 1873-1874 he was President of the Baltimore Medical Association.

1874 - George Lane Taneyhill, M.D. (1840-1916)

Dr. Taneyhill began his noteworthy career as a schoolteacher. He completed his medical degree at the University of Maryland in 1865 and served the last year of the Civil War as a surgeon with the 11th Maryland Regiment. In addition to serving as President of the Baltimore Medical Association from 1874-1875, Dr. Taneyhill was a Baltimore City School Commissioner, Vice President of the Baltimore Obstetrical and Gynaecological Society and a Founder of the Maryland Academy of Sciences. Dr. Taneyhill's *Historical Sketches of the Medical Societies of Baltimore, Md., from 1730 to 1880*, an article published in 1881, was the first formal history of professional medical organizations in Baltimore.

1875 - John T. Dickson, M.D.

A Londoner, Dr. Dickson emigrated to Baltimore and took up the study of medicine at the University of Maryland, where he received his M.D. degree in 1852. He was on the staff of Marine Hospital until 1858 and served as President of the Baltimore Medical Association. Upon retirement from a position at the Union Protestant Infirmary, Dr. Dickson returned to London.

1876 - Louis McLane Tiffany, M.D. (1844-1916)

Dr. Tiffany began his studies at the University of Cambridge in England, and received his medical degree from the University of Maryland in 1868. Over a span of 24 years, he presided over the Baltimore Medical Association, the Clinical Society of Maryland, the Medical and Chirurgical Faculty of Maryland, the American Surgical Association and the Southern Surgical and Gynaeological Association. Dr. Tiffany lectured at the Maryland Dental College and the University of Maryland and was for many years Surgeon-in-Chief to the Baltimore and Ohio Railroad.

1877 - Judson Gilman, M.D. (1818-1883)

Educated in Maine, Dr. Gilman settled in Baltimore in 1845 and was the city's Assistant Commissioner of Health for two years in the 1850's. During the Civil War, Dr. Gilman was an assistant surgeon at the prisoner of war camp at Point Lookout, in southern Maryland. He served as President of the Baltimore Medical Association, and Treasurer of the Medical and Chirurgical Faculty.

1878 - John Neff, M.D. (1832-1913)

Dr. Neff was an active member of local and state societies from his role as Founder of the Baltimore Medical Association in 1866 through his participation in the reorganization and creation of the Baltimore City Medical Society in 1904.

1879 - John Morris, M.D. (1824-1903)
Dr. Morris pursued political as well as medical careers, serving in the Maryland State Legislature from 1852-1856 and on the Baltimore City School Board from 1856-1857. Ten years later found him as a member of the Baltimore City Council, and he was the city's Postmaster from 1857-1861. His medical career officially began when he was admitted to the Medical and Chirurgical Faculty by examination (having taken just a single course at Washington Medical College) in 1845. He went on to study at Bellevue Medical College in New York where he received his medical degree, and was President of many Baltimore organizations, including the Baltimore Medical Association, the Maryland Inebriate Asylum, the Pathological Society of Baltimore, the Medical and Chirurgical Faculty of Maryland and the state Lunacy Commission. In 1879, Dr. Morris was Vice-President of the American Medical Association. During the deadly yellow fever epidemic in Norfolk, Virginia, Dr. Morris volunteered his services and was awarded a gold medal by Norfolk citizens.

1880 - John Francis Monmonier, M.D. (1813-1894)
The long and distinguished career of Dr. Monmonier began when he became a student at the University of Maryland in 1834. While still at school he served as a City Councilman in his native Baltimore, then became School Commissioner and served out his public service years as President of the School Board. Dr. Monmonier joined the faculties of the Washington University School of Medicine in physiology as well as diseases of women and children. He was President of the Medical and Chirurgical Faculty from 1875-1876.

1881 - James A. Steuart, M.D. (1828-1903)
Both son and grandson of prominent Baltimore physicians, Dr. Steuart received his medical degree from the University of Maryland in 1850. He was a Founder and President of the Epidemiological Society of Baltimore, presided over the Baltimore Pathological Society from 1874-1875 and stood three terms as Vice President of the Medical and Chirurgical Faculty. For many years, Dr. Steuart was the Commissioner of Health for Baltimore City.

1882 - Christopher Frederick Johnston, M.D. (1822-1891)
In 1844, Dr. Johnston received his M.D. degree from the University of Maryland, having studied under Dr. John Buckler. He was a Founder of the Maryland Medical Institute, lectured there beginning in 1847, and remained in academics with professorships at the Baltimore Dental College and his alma mater. Dr. Johnston was a Founder of the Baltimore Pathological Society. He went on to become Vice President of the Medical and Chirurgical Faculty in 1875 and President the following year. He served as President of the Maryland Academy of Sciences from 1885-1887. The author of

Ashurst's Encyclopedia of Surgery, a textbook on plastic surgery and skin grafting, Dr. Johnston was on the surgical staffs of Hebrew Hospital and Johns Hopkins Hospital. He was remembered as "An accomplished gentleman, an expert artist and microscopist, and a skillful surgeon."

1883 - John Summerfield Conrad, M.D. (1836-1896)
Dr. Conrad received his pharmacy degree from the Maryland College of Pharmacy in 1860 before going on to study medicine at the National Medical College in Washington and graduating two years later. He served in the Confederate Army during the Civil War as an assistant surgeon, and returned to Baltimore to take up a staff position at the Baltimore Infirmary (later University Hospital), and moved on to the staff at The Marine Hospital. His academic career included a Professorship at Washington University College of Medicine. In addition to presiding over the Baltimore Medical Association, he was Superintendent at The Maryland Hospital for the Insane (Spring Grove) and Matley Hill Sanitarium in Baltimore County.

1884 - Edmund George Waters, M.D. (1830-?)
When he was called to service in the Union Army in 1861, Dr. Waters was the President of the Young Men's Christian Association in Baltimore. At the war's conclusion he returned to Baltimore and took up a post as Professor of Natural Science at Baltimore City College. Before settling in Cambridge, Maryland in 1885, Dr. Waters was President of the Baltimore Medical Association and a Founder of the Medical and Surgical Society of Baltimore. While in Dorchester County, Maryland, Dr. Waters practiced medicine and was a member of the Maryland House of Delegates. He received his M.D. degree from the University of Maryland in 1853, a student of Nathan Ryno Smith.

1885 - Joseph Tait Smith, Jr., M.D. (1850-1930)
After completing his medical education in 1872 at the University of Maryland, Dr. Smith taught Medical Jurisprudence as well as Therapeutics at the Women's Medical College in Baltimore. From there he went to his medical alma mater and lectured in Hygiene and Medical Jurisprudence.

1886 - William Frederick Amelung Kemp, M.D. (1849-?)
Dr. Kemp, son of a Frederick, Maryland physician, graduated from the University of Maryland School of Medicine in 1872 and became an Attending Physician at the Union Protestant Infirmary (now Union Memorial Hospital). He served as Treasurer of the state medical Faculty for 15 years beginning in 1883.

1887 - Isaac Edmonson Atkinson, M.D. (1846-1906)
Dr. Atkinson's long career began when he earned his M.D. degree from the University of Maryland in 1865. He held positions on the faculty at the University, lecturing in Dermatology and Pathology. He was Dean of the University from 1890-1893, and President of the Clinical Society of Maryland. Dr. Atkinson presided over the state Faculty in 1888 while also serving as President of the American Dermatological Society.

1888 -Thomas Benjamin Evans, M.D. (1832-1891)
In 1853, Dr. Evans received his medical degree from Washington University after working as a drug store clerk. He spent the Civil War as surgeon to the Baltimore City Guards, and after the war became Professor of Ophthalmology and Pathology at Baltimore University. He was President of the Baltimore Medical and Surgical Society from 1873-1874 and again for one year beginning in 1880, and he served as Vice President of the American Medical Association for one year. His extensive medical articles included "The Relationship Between Pharmacists and Doctors, "Aims of Medical Thought," and "The Relationship Between Diphtheria and Scarlatina."

1889 - Joseph Lowrie Ingle, M.D. (1846-1914)
Educated at the University of Virginia and the University of New York, where he received his M.D. degree in 1871, Dr. Ingle was President of the Baltimore Medical Association from 1888-1889, and President of the Maryland Board of Medical Examiners in 1896.

1890 - Thomas A. Ashby, M.D. (1848-1916)
Virginian Dr. Ashby came to Baltimore in 1873 and in 1877 founded the *Maryland Medical Journal*. In addition to a position on the faculty of the University of Maryland, he founded the Woman's Medical College of Baltimore in 1882. Dr. Ashby was considered a pioneer in the study of women's medical issues, and served as the President of the Baltimore Gynaecological and Obstetrical Society in 1897. He also held various offices in the state medical Faculty.

1891 - John Wesley Chambers, M.D. (1856-?)
Dr. Chambers enjoyed a long career as lecturer, demonstrator and professor at his alma mater, the College of Physicians and Surgeons, in Baltimore. He also lectured at the Baltimore College of Dental Surgery, and was President of the Baltimore Medical Association and the state Faculty.

1892 - Jacob Edwin Michael, M.D. (1848-1895)
In 1871, Dr. Michael received his baccalaureate degree from Princeton, after which he studied medicine at the University of Maryland. He rose through the ranks of the faculty there and served

as Dean from 1886-1890 and again from 1893-1895. He had a distinguished career as a leader of many professional societies, as President of both the Baltimore Medical Association and the Clinical Society, as well as Vice President and President of the Medical and Chirurgical Faculty. Dr. Michael also presided over the alumni associations at both of his alma maters, Princeton and the University of Maryland.

1893 - David Streett, M.D. (1855-1915)
After receiving his baccalaureate degree from Loyola College in Maryland, Dr. Streett went on to study medicine and later serve on the faculty of the College of Physicians and Surgeons. He presided over both the Baltimore Medical Association and the Medical and Surgical Society (1891-1892), and held the post of Vice President at the Medical and Chirurgical Faculty for the same years. He served one term on the First Branch of the Baltimore City Council.

1894 - Hampson Hubert Biedler, M.D. (1854-?)
After receiving his M.D. degree at the University of Maryland, Dr. Biedler returned to his home in Rappahannock County, Virginia to practice medicine. In 1882 he returned to Baltimore to take up posts on the faculties of the Baltimore Medical College and Baltimore University, where he was Professor of Diseases of Women.

1895 - Randolph Winslow, M.D. (1852-1937)
Dr. Winslow enjoyed a long career on the faculty of the University of Maryland, where he received his medical degree in 1873. He was a Professor of Anatomy and Clinical Surgery at the University, at Baltimore Polyclinic he taught Operative Surgery and Topographic Anatomy, and he was on the faculty at the Women's Medical College of Baltimore. Dr. Winslow was Vice President of the Medical and Chirurgical Faculty for one year beginning in 1896.

1896 - James Edward Gibbons, M.D. (1844-1901)
Dr. Gibbons attended lectures at the University of Maryland and Washington University College of Medicine, where he received his medical degree in 1868. His early practice was in New Windsor, Maryland, but he returned to Baltimore in 1875, where he became a vaccine physician.

1897 - John Bushrod Schwatka, M.D. (1861-1926)
Dr. Schwatka may be the only physician who also served as Sheriff for the City of Baltimore (1899-1901). He earned his M.D. Degree from the University of Maryland in 1882, practiced briefly in Delaware, and after became a member of the faculty of the Baltimore Medical College, lecturing on Anatomy. After the merger of the Baltimore Medical Association and the Medical and Surgical Society of Baltimore, he served as President in 1897.

In 1897, the Baltimore Medical Association and the Medical and Surgical Society of Baltimore merged. The group adopted a new name: The Baltimore Medical and Surgical Association.

1898 - John I. Pennington, M.D. (1842-1924)
Dr. Pennington was on the staff at the Presbyterian Eye, Ear and Throat Hospital in Baltimore and was the President of the Baltimore Medical and Surgical Association. He received his M.D. degree from the University of Maryland in 1869. When he passed away, the Sun noted that he was "One of the oldest and most widely known general practitioners in Baltimore. He was the type of days gone by, suave, courteous, kindly, an old-time family doctor."

1899 - C. Urban Smith, M.D. (?-1945)

1900 - Cary Breckinridge Gamble, Jr., M.D. (1862-?)
Dr. Gamble received his M.D. degree from the University of Maryland in 1887, and was a Professor of Clinical Medicine at the College of Physicians and Surgeons in Baltimore.

1901 - Charles Geraldus Hill, M.D.
In 1890, Dr. Hill received a medical degree from the Washington University in Baltimore. He was President of the Medical and Chirurgical Faculty of Maryland from 1895-1896. His academic career was spent entirely at the University of Maryland, where he lectured on nervous and mental disorders, eventually becoming a full Professor. Dr. Hill also presided over the Baltimore County Medical Society in 1898. An amateur astronomer, in 1881, he discovered a comet that is named after him.

1902 - J. Lowrie Ingle, M.D.
(See 1889)

1903 - Edward L. Whitney, M.D. (1870-?)
After receiving his baccalaureate degree from Oberlin College, Dr. Whitney continued his education at the University of Maryland, where he received a medical degree in 1895. He studied in Berlin for several years and returned to Baltimore to take up a post at Maryland General Hospital. He became an Associate Professor in Physiological Chemistry at the University of Maryland, and is the author of *A Laboratory Manual of Clinical Pathology*.

1904 - J.M. Craighill, M.D. (1857-?)
After receiving his medical degree from the University of Maryland in 1882, Dr. Craighill took up a post as Resident Physician at Bayview Hospital. He began his academic career as a Demonstrator of Anatomy at the University of Maryland, and in 1900 became an Assistant Professor of Clinical Medicine.

Other pre-1904 society Presidents of distinction not included above:

Augustus F. Erich, M.D., Founding President of the East Baltimore Medical Society (1837-1886)
In 1856, Dr. Erich emigrated to Baltimore from Prussia and after receiving his medical degree from the University of Maryland in 1861 immediately became active in the professional medical community. He invented an "automatic draining apparatus" which, powered by the flow of water from a fire hydrant, pumped water from Baltimore cellars. The pump was credited with having preserved many Baltimoreans from infection during the 1866 Asiatic Cholera epidemic, and he was granted a patent the same year. He became a member of the first State Board of Medical Examiners in 1867, having championed legislation "to draw up a law for the suppression of quackery and criminal abortion," which passed in Annapolis in 1866. In 1871 he founded the Medical and Surgical Society of Baltimore (originally the East Baltimore Medical Society) and two years later edited *Baltimore Physician and Surgeon*. He also presided over the Pathological Society of Baltimore, the Medical and Chirurgical Faculty, the Clinical Society of Baltimore and the Maryland Academy of Sciences. A Founder of Maryland Women's Hospital, Dr. Erich invented the self-retaining vaginal speculum. His daughter, Louise Erich, M.D., became a physician specializing in diseases of the eye.

John D. Blake, M.D. (1853-1920)
In 1875, Dr. Blake received his degree from the College of Physicians and Surgeons in Baltimore, and went on to become a city vaccine physician until 1881. While a faculty member at the Baltimore Medical College and a Baltimore City Councilman, he also was President of the Medical and Surgical Society, and from 1893-1894 was Secretary of the state medical Faculty.

Baltimore City Medical Society (The year in which the physician was President appears before the name):

1904 - Harry Friedenwald, M.D. (1864-1950)
Dr. Friedenwald combined his medical career with an equally-important career as a leader in the Zionist movement. Graduating from the College of Physicians and Surgeons with a medical degree in 1886, he went on to lecture on diseases of the eye and ear at his alma mater. Following a year as Vice President of the state Medical and Chirurgical Faculty, Dr. Friedenwald became President of the newly-reorganized Baltimore City Medical Society in 1904, and

served as President again in 1913. His legacy is not only medical, but historic. In 1930 he presented his extensive collection of art and manuscripts, including important and rare books on medicine, to the University of Palestine.

1905 -Henry Ottrage (Ottridge) Reik, M.D. (1868-1938)

With degrees from the Maryland College of Pharmacy and the University of Maryland, Dr. Reik became an eye and ear surgeon and author of three important books: *Treatment of Diseases of the Ear, Nose and Throat*, *Surgical Pathology*, and *Safeguarding the Special Senses*. After 25 years of practice, Dr. Reik lost the use of his right hand in 1916 and was forced to retire.

"I sometimes feel rather blue when I look ahead and see that I am not going to be able to realize my aspirations in life..."

WILLIAM HENRY WELCH, M.D. (1850-1934)

The physician who in 1880 looked upon his professional life in America with disappointment ended his career by being heralded as "our greatest statesman in the field of public health" by President Herbert Hoover. Connecticut-born Dr. Welch never served as the President of a Baltimore medical society (though he was President of the Medical and Chirurgical Faculty of Maryland from 1891-1892). He was, however, in addition to being one of the city's most celebrated physicians, the President of the Board of Directors of the Rockefeller Medical Research Institute, the Maryland Public Health Association and Dean of the Medical Faculty at Johns Hopkins University. His name is memorialized in Baltimore medical circles, indeed in medical circles around the world, as one of the "Big Four" on whose reputation Johns Hopkins University Medical School and Hospital was founded.

Receiving his medical degree at the age of 25 at the Columbia University College of Physicians and Surgeons, Dr. Welch went on to study at Western Reserve, Harvard and Yale (where, curiously enough, he served briefly as a tutor in Greek). His first medical teaching position was at the Bellevue Hospital Medical College, where he lectured on anatomy and general pathology. It was while at Bellevue, working in a laboratory that consisted of three bare rooms with kitchen tables and "fully twenty-five dollars in laboratory equipment" that he bemoaned the state of research. "There is no opportunity in this country," he wrote, "and it seems probable that there never will be."

Opportunity knocked when President Gilman asked him in 1886 to join the staff at Johns Hopkins University, seven years before the medical school opened. As plans for the medical school developed, it was Dr. Welch's insistence that Dr. William Osler be named Professor of Medicine that resulted in the Canadian's appointment (the first choice was an English physician, but Welch prevailed). Drs. William S. Halsted and Howard Atwood Kelly joined the faculty, and the school was to begin with the four most influential medical men in the nation at its head.

Dr. Welch became the university's public health authority early in his career at Hopkins. He was nominated to the State Board of Health in 1898 and two years later was its President, a post he held for 22 years. He was instrumental in the founding of the National Tuberculosis Association. In 1914, in spite of significant political opposition, Dr. Welch's impassioned plea to the Maryland legislature that a statewide network of ten sanitary districts be created because of the deplorable sanitary conditions in rural areas led to passage of the important Bill. He fought for chlorination of the city water supply and for a milk ordinance that ended the threat of milk-borne typhoid.

Recognizing that Baltimore desperately needed a communicable disease hospital, Dr. Welch's advocacy led to the establishment of Sydenham Hospital in 1909, then a small facility next to Bayview. In 1924, when demand had long since outstripped the old building, his leadership resulted in a modern, new Sydenham at Lake Montebello.

A fixture at local medical society meetings, Dr. Welch advocated for every major public health initiative from the establishment of the Baltimore City Medical Society in 1904 to his death. During the Water Loan effort in 1908 to upgrade the city's water and sanitary facilities, he lobbied intensely about the need for clean water (even though he suspected that milk was more to blame for typhoid's scourge) and the Society supported the measure. He was back again to urge the passage of milk regulations.

A Welch biographer, Dr. Harvey Cushing (also a Society President) wrote of the doctor for the Hoover memorial on his 80th birthday, that "to have done so much, in so many ways and to have aroused no shadow of enmity or envy, betokens not only unselfishness of purpose but also that fineness of character which always has been an inspiration to mankind."

1906 - William Sydney Thayer, M.D. (1864-1932)

Dr. Thayer received his training at Harvard, where he earned his medical degree in 1889. Well known in international medical circles, Dr. Thayer was the author of *The Malarial Fevers of Baltimore: An Analysis of 616 Cases of Malarial Fever*. During the First World War he was Chief Medical Officer of the American Expeditionary Forces in France, rising to the rank of Brigadier General. He served on the faculty of Johns Hopkins University, where he was the successor to Sir William Osler, M.D. Seldom seen without a flower in his buttonhole, Dr. Thayer was also known for his aristocratic carriage (and his absent-mindedness).

1907 - Archibald Cunningham Harrison, M.D. (1864-1926)

Dr. Harrison came to Baltimore from his home in Virginia, completed his medical education begun at the University of Virginia with a degree from the University of Maryland in 1887, and pursued an academic career on the faculties of the Women's Medical College and the College of Physicians and Surgeons. Dr. Harrison was also

President of the Somerset County (Pennsylvania) Medical Association.

1908 - Wilmer Brinton, M.D. (1853-?)
When Dr. Brinton became President of the Baltimore City Medical Society, it was his second stint presiding over a local organization. From 1879-1880 he was President of the Medical and Surgical Society of Baltimore, and after that Vice President of the state Faculty. Following receipt of his medical degree from the University of Maryland in 1876, Dr. Brinton joined the faculty of the Baltimore Medical College as Professor of Obstetrics. "It is impossible to estimate the number of infants named after him," his obituary writer reported.

1909 - Jacob Henry Hartman, M.D. (1847-1916)
Dr. Hartman was a student of Dr. Nathan Ryno Smith, one of the nation's most esteemed medical men in the mid-1800's, and received his M.D. degree from the University of Maryland in 1869. He went on to study in Paris, Berlin, Vienna and London before returning to become a lecturer at Washington University in Baltimore. A Founder of the Baltimore Eye, Ear and Throat Charity Hospital, Dr. Hartman was also Vice President of the American Laryngological Association.

1910 - Harvey Williams Cushing, M.D. (1869-1939)
After receiving his M.D. from Harvard in 1895, Dr. Cushing trained in surgery at Johns Hopkins under Dr. William Halsted. After several years traveling in Europe, Dr. Cushing returned to the United States where he became well known for his work in neurosurgery, including standardization of neurosurgical technique and the classification of brain tumors. In 1912 he became Professor of Surgery at the Harvard Medical School and authored an important volume on the pituitary gland. Dr. Cushing went on to become the first Chief of Surgery at Boston's Peter Bent Brigham Hospital. In 1932, he went to Yale as the Sterling Professor in Neurology. Cushing's Disease, an endocrine disorder, was named after him, and he is remembered as the foremost neurosurgeon of his day. He developed many of the techniques and procedures used today in surgery of the brain and spinal cord and was one of the first surgeons to employ x-ray technology in the operating room. Dr. Cushing established the Hunterian Laboratory of Experimental Medicine at Hopkins and wrote a Pulitzer Prize winning biography of Dr. William Osler.

1911 - Arthur Marriott Shipley, M.D. (1878-1955)
"King Arthur," as Dr. Shipley was known among his colleagues, graduated from the University of Maryland School of Medicine in

1902 and later reorganized the surgical service at his alma mater while acting as Chief Surgeon. An author of more than 80 articles in professional journals, Dr. Shipley also served with the U.S. Army during World War I. He was President of the Baltimore City Medical Society in 1911, and in 1937 rose to the Presidency of the Medical and Chirurgical Faculty of Maryland.

1912 - Robert Wilkinson Johnson, M.D. (1854-1930)
In 1912, Dr. Johnson became President of the Baltimore City Medical Society. He had practiced medicine for over 3 decades by then, having been granted his medical degree at the University of Pennsylvania in 1879. In 1894 he assumed the Presidency of the state medical Faculty, was on the faculty of the Baltimore Medical College and on the surgical staff at Church Home and Infirmary. Dr. Johnson also held posts as Surgeon at Maryland Steel Company (later Bethlehem Steel) and the Baltimore Mutual Life and Annuity Company, and the Surgeon General of Maryland.

1913 - Harry Friedenwald, M.D.
(See 1904)

1914 - Thomas Richardson Brown, M.D. (1872-1950)
Son of a President of the Medical and Surgical Society of Baltimore, Dr. Brown presided over the Baltimore City Medical Society in 1914 and the American Gastroenterological Association in 1919. He received both his baccalaureate and his medical degrees from Johns Hopkins University (1897), went on to staff positions at Hopkins and the Johns Hopkins Dispensary and taught at the College of Physicians and Surgeons.

1915 - Charles E. Sadtler, M.D. (1851-1927)
Dr, Sadtler received his M.D. degree from the University of Maryland in 1873, after which he became Dispensary Physician at his alma mater.

1916 - Charles Hampson Jones, M.D. (1858-1932)
With his new undergraduate degree from Johns Hopkins University, Dr. Jones continued his medical education at the University of Edinburgh (1883). By 1886 he was back in Baltimore, teaching physiology at the Women's Medical College and later at the College of Physicians and Surgeons. Dr. Jones also had a distinguished public health career, having served as Health Commissioner at both city and state levels. He was an early advocate of the pasteurization of milk and improvement of the city's water supply system. Unafraid of controversy, Dr. Jones enforced compulsory vaccination city-wide against diphtheria and smallpox, ending fumigation in Baltimore as a preventive technique. He presided over the Baltimore City Medical Society in 1916 and the state Faculty in 1917.

1917 - Thomas Stephen Cullen, M.D. (1868-1953)
In 1900, Dr. Cullen began a decades-long effort to educate the public about cancer with the publication of his book *Cancer of the Uterus*. His 1913 article on the same subject in the popular *Ladies Home Journal* raised the ire of a medical community that was still skeptical of public education measures. The Johns Hopkins Nurses' Alumni Magazine, in a 1947 article, called him a "pioneer for public education in cancer control." A native Canadian, He graduated from Toronto University in 1890 and by 1892 was on the staff of Johns Hopkins Hospital.

1918 - Randolph Winslow, M.D. (1852-1937)
Dr. Winslow's career includes several pioneering surgeries. According to the *Maryland Medical Journal*, he introduced antiseptic surgery into practice in Maryland (photos of the surgery at Johns Hopkins as late as the 1890's show physicians and nurses with neither gloves nor masks, and both attendants and bystanders with bare heads). He was the first surgeon in Maryland to resect the pylorus for carcinoma, performed an early vaginal hysterectomy (1888) and was the first surgeon to resect intestines following a gunshot wound. After receiving a medical degree from the University of Maryland in 1873, Dr. Winslow began a 30-year academic career there and at the Women's Medical College, in Baltimore, of which he was a Founder. He was Vice President of the Medical and Chirurgical Faculty from 1896-1897, President of the state Faculty in 1914.

1919 - Guy Leroy Hunner, M.D. (1868-1957)
A member of the first graduating class of the Johns Hopkins University School of Medicine (1897), Dr. Hunner coupled medicine with an avocation in farming and landscape gardening. A urologist, he "rediscovered" stricture of the ureter as a surgical complication (the original discovery, by Hopkins surgeon Dr. Howard A. Kelly, having been lost). A staff physician at Hebrew Hospital, Dr. Hunner was awarded the "Research Medal" by the Southern Medical Association in 1950. "He was reserved in manner, with the courtliness of the old school."

1920 - Harvey Brinton Stone, M.D. (1882-1977)
Dr. Stone is well known for having developed revolutionary methods of glandular tissue transplant from donor to recipient in the 1930's. During World War I he served in France with the Johns Hopkins Hospital unit, and after his return from Europe he became a researcher and Associate Professor Emeritus at Hopkins. He volunteered during the Second World War, when he was a member of the National Board of Procurement and Assignment Service, which recruited physicians to aid in the war effort.

1921 - Harvey Grant Beck, M.D. (1870-1951)
Internist Dr. Beck received his medical degree from the College of Physicians and Surgeons in 1896, after first having graduated from the University of Maryland School of Pharmacy. He did extensive research work on carbon monoxide poisoning and diseases of the stomach, and was President of the American Therapeutic Society.

1922 - Thomas Barnes Futcher, M.D. (1871-1938)
While on the faculty at Johns Hopkins, endocrinologist Dr. Futcher frequently took students to the circus sideshow, which he called the "Greatest Endocrine Clinic on Earth." A Canadian, he received his medical degree from the University of Toronto in 1893, and served as a Lieutenant Colonel in the Canadian Army Medical Corps during World War I. In Baltimore, Dr. Futcher became a close associate of Dr. William Osler. He served on the faculty and staff at Hopkins throughout his career, and presided over the Baltimore City Medical Society. Recognized as one of the country's leading diagnosticians, Dr. Futcher was noted for metabolism research.

1923 - Alexius McGlannan, Jr., M.D. (1872-1940)
A native Baltimorean and son of a pharmacist, Dr. McGlannan began his medical studies at the Maryland College of Pharmacy, where he received a degree in 1890. In 1895, he earned a medical degree from the College of Physicians and Surgeons in Baltimore and went on to staff positions at City Hospital, St. Joseph's Hospital and St. Elizabeth's Home for Children. On the faculties of the University of Maryland and Johns Hopkins University, Dr. McGlannan was also Chief of Surgery at Mercy Hospital.

1924 - Gordon Wilson, M.D. (1876-1932)
In addition to presiding over the Baltimore City Medical Society, Dr. Wilson was on the faculty at the University of Maryland. He received his medical degree from the University of Virginia. In Baltimore, he was Chief of the Department of Medicine at University Hospital, Chief of the Tuberculosis Department at Baltimore City Hospitals, and served on the Maryland Tuberculosis Commission.

1925 - Charles French Blake, M.D. (1866-1948)
Dr. Blake studied medicine at the University of Ohio and received his medical degree from the College of Physicians and Surgeons in 1893. He was on the staff at City Hospital immediately after his graduation and worked as visiting physician at the Bayview Asylum. He continued his relationship with his alma mater as a Demonstrating Surgeon and later as a lecturer in anatomy. Dr. Blake's obituary read: "Another horse and buggy doctor was taken from us today when Charles F. Blake died," though it went on to

note that he was one of the first physicians in Baltimore to purchase an automobile to make house calls.

1926 - William Topping Watson, M.D. (1851-1926)
In 1891, Canadian Dr. Watson received an M.D. degree from the University of Maryland after study at Johns Hopkins University. His academic career began as an Associate Professor in public health and hygiene at Baltimore Medical College, and Professor of Therapeutics at the University of Maryland. Shortly after having taken up the Presidency of the Baltimore City Medical Society in 1926, Dr. Watson died of septicemia.

1927 - Edward Henderson Richardson, M.D. (1877-1971)
Unexpectedly becoming President of Baltimore City Medical Society after the unexpected death of his predecessor, Dr. Richardson remained in office through 1927. His first professional degree was in accounting and after completing studies at the Eastman Business College he came to Baltimore, and eventually received his M.D. degree from Johns Hopkins University in 1905. Gynecologist Dr. Richardson is known for the Richardson Composite Operation, to repair cystoceles.

1928 - Joseph Albert Chatard, M.D. (1879-1956)
Dr. Chatard followed his father, grandfather and great-grandfather into medicine and received his own degree from Johns Hopkins University in 1903. For several years in the 1920's the Baltimore City Medical Society met at the Chatard Building on Maryland Avenue, where he had his private practice. Dr. Chatard was President of the Baltimore City Medical Society in 1928, and in 1932 held the same position at the state Faculty after having already been Secretary and Treasurer.

1929 - Joseph Colt Bloodgood, M.D. (1867-1935)
Receiving his medical degree from the University of Pennsylvania in 1891, Dr. Bloodgood went on to a long and distinguished career, primarily in cancer research. In Baltimore, Dr. Bloodgood became Chief of Surgery at St. Agnes Hospital after a 13-year career as a surgeon at Johns Hopkins. Dr. Bloodgood was internationally renowned leader in the fight against cancer, and won a gold medal in 1924 from the Radiological Society of North America for his work in studying bone malignancies.

1930 - Charles Bagley, M.D. (1882-1957)
Dr. Bagley received his medical degree from the Washington University School of Medicine in Baltimore in 1904 and did his neurosurgery residency in Boston under Dr. Harvey Cushing. Dr. Bagley, upon his return to Baltimore, became Chief of the Neurosurgery Department at the University of Maryland. During

World War I, Dr. Bagley was assigned to the Office of the United States Surgeon General, where he established a section on head surgery for the Army. He went to Europe as a consultant, and upon his return was assigned to the Fort McHenry Army Hospital. In civilian life, Dr. Bagley resumed research at the Phipps Clinic and served on the staff at St. Agnes Hospital.

1931 - Louis Philip Hamburger, M.D. (1873-?)
Dr. Hamburger earned his medical degree with the first graduating class of Johns Hopkins University in 1897.

1932 - Dean DeWitt Lewis, M.D. (1874-1941)
Dr. Lewis, during his long years at Johns Hopkins Hospital, published a serialized book entitled *The Lewis Practice of Surgery*, which was purchased by subscription and arrived pre-punched for a looseleaf binder. He was granted an M.D. degree in 1897, succeeded Dr. William Halsted at Hopkins as Chair of the Department of Surgery and remained as Chair for 13 years. His years at Hopkins were interrupted by World War I. As Lieutenant Colonel in the Army Medical Corps, he spent most of the war years at emergency hospitals at the Front, in particular as Chief of Surgery at Service Evacuation Hospital Number Five. For his military contributions he received the Distinguished Service Medal in 1922: "During operations on the Marne, in St. Mihiel, the Meuse-Argonne and the Ypres offensives, by his tireless energy, organizing ability and unusual surgical skill, Dr. Lewis demonstrated that war wounds could be operated upon in large numbers in front-line hospitals with limited personnel." One of his most important discoveries was the "cable transplant," a method of joining two severed nerve ends that are so impaired that the intervening sections of nerve tissue were destroyed. Dr. Lewis was the President of the American Medical Association in 1933.

1933 - Julius Friedenwald, M.D. (1866-1941)
In 1890, Dr. Friedenwald received his medical degree from the College of Physicians and Surgeons in Baltimore, after which he remained in the faculty as Associate Professor of Pathology and Clinical Professor of Diseases of the Stomach. Later in his career he served on the staff at both City Hospital and St. Agnes Hospital.

1934 - Warfield Longcope, M.D. (1877-1953)
Dr. Longcope, the great-grandson of Dr. Nathan Ryno Smith, succeeded Drs. Osler and Thayer at Johns Hopkins University. He made vital contributions to medical literature through his studies of diseases arising from protein poisoning, and by the 1940's was one of the world's leading authorities on diseases of the arteries.

"...to advance the ethical practice of medicine..."

1935 - Frank S. Lynn, M.D. (1884-1938)
Dr. Lynn was a Professor of Clinical Surgery at the University of Maryland, where he spent his entire medical academic career. In addition to presiding over the Baltimore City Medical Society, he was also President of the B&O Association of Railway Surgeons.

1936 - Charles Chauncey Windsor Judd, M.D. (1883-?)
Receiving his medical degree form Johns Hopkins University in 1911, Dr. Judd was President of the Baltimore City Medical Society in 1936, when he hosted the 13th Annual Convention of the Southern Medical Association in Baltimore.

1937 - Robert Parke Bay, M.D. (1884-1940)
Dr. Bay served on the Board of Managers of the Baltimore General Dispensary after receiving his medical degree from the University of Maryland in 1905. During World War I he taught in the Army Medical Corps at Camp Oglethorp and stayed in the military as Chief Surgeon of the Maryland National Guard.

1938 - Charles Robert Austrian, M.D. (1885-1956)
Dr. Austrian established his private practice in Baltimore after receiving his medical degree from Johns Hopkins University in 1909. Internationally known as a consultant in internal medicine, Dr. Austrian was on the faculty at Hopkins, Chief Physician at Sinai Hospital, and presided over the Johns Hopkins Medical Society and the Medical and Chirurgical Faculty.

1939 - Eugene H. Hayward, M.D. (1877-1958)
After receiving a medical degree from the Baltimore Medical College (eventually merged into the University of Maryland system), Dr. Hayward served in France during World War I with the University of Maryland unit. Upon his return, he worked on the staffs at St. Joseph's Hospital, Bon Secours Hospital, Church Home and Hospital and Mercy Hospital.

1940 - George Carroll Lockard, M.D. (1882-1949)
Dr. Lockard was President of the Baltimore City Medical Society in 1940, and in 1946 presided over the state medical Faculty. He was on the faculty of the University of Maryland as Professor of Clinical Medicine.

1941 - William Herbert Pearce, M.D. (1870-1951)
Remembered as a "great defender of the general practitioner as opposed to the specialist," Dr. Pearce graduated from the University of Maryland in 1891.

1942 - Lawrence Wharton, M.D. (1887-1974)
Dr. Wharton was a gynecologist on the staff at both Union Memorial Hospital and Johns Hopkins University.

1943 - Walter Dent Wise, M.D. (1885-1968)
Dr. Wise held positions as Professor of Surgery at the University of Maryland and Chief of Surgery at Mercy Hospital. During the Second World War, Dr. Wise was the Medical Director of the Selective Service of Maryland, and a Consulting Surgeon to the U.S. Army Third Medical Command. He received the Army Legion of Merit Award, the Army Service Medal, the World War II Victory Medal and the Selective Service Medal. After presiding over the Baltimore City Medical Society, Dr. Wise went on to become President of the state Faculty in 1951.

1944 - Thomas P. Sprunt, M.D.
With Dr. Lewellys Baker, Dr. Sprunt wrote *The Degenerative Diseases, Their Causes and Prevention*, published as part of the Johns Hopkins Public Health Series in 1925.

1945 - Louis Harriman Douglas, M.D.
Dr. Douglas was Chairman of Obstetrics at the University of Maryland.

1946 - Alfred Blalock, M.D. (1899-1964)
Dr. Blalock followed Drs. Lewis and Halsted as Chief of the Department of Surgery at Johns Hopkins Hospital and has many pioneering surgical techniques to his credit. He performed groundbreaking work in the treatment of shock, and was an early advocate for the use of plasma in transfusions. With Dr. Helen Taussig (a Baltimore City Medical Society member) he created the "blue baby" surgery to correct congenital heart disorders in newborns. His contributions were recognized in 1949, when he was awarded honors for his pioneering discoveries in vascular surgery from the International Society of Surgery, and in 1953 when he won the American Medical Association's Distinguished Service Award. Twelve years after Dr. Blalock died, Dr. Richard Ross, Dean of the Johns Hopkins University School of Medicine, said that "The astonishing progress of cardiac surgery in the last 30 years began with Blalock and Taussig."

1947 - Charles Reid Edwards, M.D. (1888-1965)
Dr Edwards was a member of the famed "Surgical Triad" at the University of Maryland, with Drs. Arthur Shipley and Frank Lynn. He graduated with an M.D. degree from the University of Maryland in 1913, and remained as Professor of Clinical Surgery, eventually rising to head of the Department of Surgery. Dr. Edwards also presided over the Medical and Chirurgical Faculty.

"It is the clinical errors that keep you humble...On the whole, though, I think I've done more good than harm."

HELEN BROOKE TAUSSIG, M.D. (1898-1986)

Surely the thousands of adults who are alive and healthy, thanks to the groundbreaking "blue baby" surgery pioneered by Dr. Helen Taussig and her colleague, Dr. Alfred Blalock, would come down on the side of good.
The 1944 discovery of a surgical technique to correct pulmonary stenosis, a condition which tints its sufferers' lips and fingers blue because of inadequate flow of blood from the heart to the lungs, made Dr. Taussig a household name. The procedure, which alters the course of a major artery by connecting it to the artery going to the lungs (in effect giving the blood a "second chance" for oxygenation) was Dr. Taussig's idea. For it, she was named "The Outstanding Woman in Science for 1948" by the Associated Press, given an 1947 award by the Women's National Press Club, the American Heart Association's Award of Merit in 1953, named a Chevalier in the French Legion of Honor in 1947, and recipient of an Eleanor Roosevelt Achievement Award in 1957.

The brilliant heart surgeon who would go on to head the Cardiac Clinic of the Harriet Lane Home at Hopkins for 23 years was denied an internship in medicine at Hopkins following her 1927 graduation. Another woman had already been admitted, and the University would admit two female practitioners into the same specialty. She chose instead an internship in pediatrics. "She grew up in an era when some people said it didn't pay to educate women...It paid to educate Helen Brooke Taussig...She never married, never had children, but her work helped to save the lives of thousands of babies and save thousands of others from revolting deformity," biographer Jeanne Stevenson said of her in *Notable American Women*. Had she gone to another hospital for her internship, Hopkins would almost certainly have been denied her 39 years as Professor, and the notoriety she brought to the University.

In 1962, Dr. Taussig received a letter from a colleague in Germany reporting inexplicable deformities in babies that he believed resulting from their mothers' having taken a sleeping pill during pregnancy. Intrigued, she went to Germany to investigate and became the first American physician to report on the horrible effects of Thalidomide. Disturbing pictures of children with malformed limbs filled American newspapers, though Dr. Taussig's work prevented millions of American mothers from making the same mistake. For this, President Lyndon Johnson presented her with a Medal of Freedom in 1964, the highest honor a President can bestow upon a civilian. The next year she became the first female President of the American Heart Association. She was also a passionate lobbyist and advocate for the freedom of researchers to operate without government interference, and for the Medicare program. The *Evening Sun*, in 1963, called her "a persistent scientist with regard to research...a stubborn fighter against federal law that she considers detrimental to the cause of medicine," referring to her fight against the anti-vivisection society initiative to stop the use of dogs in medical research. She spoke against socialized medicine. For Medicare, however, she had other opinions: "The AMA...has done nothing but oppose the President's plan...It is inevitable that a system of private practice and a modified form of socialized medicine will be worked out. The handwriting is on the wall," she said in 1963.

After receiving the AMA's Scientific Achievement Award in 1977, Dr. Taussig was honored by the Baltimore City Medical Society, of which she was a longtime member (but never President). This was her 23rd important award, and counting her 19 honorary degrees, it is easy to understand why the Society was "honored by having such a distinguished physician and humanitarian as a member."

1948 - John T. King, M.D. (1889-1979)
During Dr. King's presidency of the Baltimore City Medical Society, the revolutionary decision to admit African American physicians as full members was made. His social activism and advocacy continued when in 1958 he became one of the first physicians to speak out in favor of treatment of narcotics addicts rather than imprisonment. Dr. King, an internist at Johns Hopkins Hospital and the Walter Reed Medical Center, introduced the general use of electrocardiograms in Baltimore and testing for thyroid disease. His autobiography was an outspoken description on the loss of physicians' autonomy as medicine became more and more under the control of insurance companies.

1949 - Albert Elias Goldstein, M.D. (1887-1966)
Dr. Goldstein received his M.D. degree from the College of Physicians and Surgeons in 1912. His specialty was general surgery and genito-urinary surgery, and he organized and directed the Hoffberger Urological Research Laboratory at Sinai Hospital. In addition to presiding over the Baltimore City Medical Society, he was also president of the state medical Faculty and the Mid-Atlantic Urological Society. Dr. Goldstein was an Associate Professor of Urology at the University of Maryland. With the assistance of Dr. Seymour W. Rubin, he perfected the artificial bladder in 1947.

1950 - John Miller Turpin Finney, M.D. (1894-1969)
Dr. Finney followed his Harvard-educated father into medicine and onto the staff at the Johns Hopkins Hospital. The elder Dr. Finney was an early advocate of expanding access to health care across racial lines and an ardent supporter of fundraising efforts to secure the financial future of Provident Hospital After receiving his M.D. from Hopkins in 1919, the younger Dr. Finney enlisted and worked at the Johns Hopkins Base Hospital in France. Upon his return, he became a surgeon at Hopkins and later at Union Memorial Hospital. Over his career he published 20 professional papers.

1951 - Louis Krause, M.D. (1896-1975)
When not lecturing on General Medicine, Clinical Medicine or the History of Medicine at the University of Maryland, Dr. Krause

could be found at one of the telescopes in the observatory he had built onto his home. He received his medical degree from the University in 1917, and with the degree he received the Faculty Gold Medal, the highest honor given to graduates. Dr. Krause served in both World Wars, at the front in World War I with the American Expeditionary Forces and as Chief of Medical Services at Walter Reed Medical Center during World War II. After the first war he returned to Baltimore and became the Chief of Medical Services at Lutheran Hospital. An interest in ancient diseases led to his being invited to participate in an archaeological expedition to Oman and Saudi Arabia in 1950, where he organized free clinics. Dr. Krause also journeyed to Egypt to study the history of disease revealed by excavations of mummies. A lifelong bachelor, Dr. Krause devoted much of his time to missionary work.

1952 - Samuel McLanahan, M.D. (1901-1961)
Having earned his M.D. degree at Johns Hopkins University in 1927, Dr. McLanahan served as a surgeon on the staffs of Johns Hopkins Hospital, Union Memorial Hospital and Women's Hospital. In 1951, at the special request of the government of Kuwait, Dr. McLanahan traveled to the Middle East to care for a member of the ruling family, Sheikh Shayks Subah al Naser.

1953 - Wetherbee Fort, M.D. (1895-1968)
Dr. Fort, in addition to presiding over the Baltimore City Medical Society, was an internist and a member of the University of Maryland Board of Trustees. He was Chief of Surgery at Union Memorial Hospital. The first coronary care unit at Union Memorial was named after Dr. Fort.

1954 - Lewis P. Gundry, M.D.
An internist at the private Gundry Sanitorium, in Catonsville, Maryland, Dr. Gundry also taught physical diagnosis. During World War II, he served with the University of Maryland Unit in the Pacific. In 1960, Dr. Gundry was tapped to head Maryland's first Commission on Alcoholism.

1955 - Amos Ralph Koontz, M.D. (1890-1965)
The politically outspoken Dr. Koontz was Chairman of the Committee on Public Medical Education for many years before becoming President of the Baltimore City Medical Society. "Famous Amos," as he was known to his students, was noted for hernia repairs when he was surgeon at Johns Hopkins Hospital. He was especially proud of his military career, being the only physician to serve with the Johns Hopkins University unit in both World Wars. Immediately after receiving his medical degree from Hopkins in 1918, Dr. Koontz enlisted and served in military hospitals in France. Before the outbreak of the Second World War, Dr. Koontz was

THE BALTIMORE CITY MEDICAL SOCIETY - A History

Medical Director of the Selective Service, and served in the South Pacific until the war's end.

1956 - Grant Eben Ward, M.D. (1896-1958)
In 1921, Dr. Ward received his M.D. degree from the University of Maryland and he continued at the University as a surgeon, as well as serving a similar role on the staff at Johns Hopkins Hospital. Though he suffered from proximal paralysis of one arm he could still practice surgery and radium therapy. Dr. Ward is credited with pioneering efforts in oncology.

1957 - Francis Joseph Geraghty, M.D. (1898-1958)
Beginning his medical career with a degree from the University of Maryland in 1926, Dr. Geraghty went on to teaching positions at the University, Chief of Medicine at St. Joseph's Hospital, and Chief of Staff at Bon Secours Hospital. He was Secretary of the Baltimore City Medical Society for 7 years before accepting its Presidency.

1958 - Whitmer B. Firor, M.D. (1902-1979)
Dr. Firor was Chief of Radiology at Union Memorial Hospital, where he practiced for 35 years. His medical degree was conferred by Johns Hopkins in 1927. He joined the Johns Hopkins unit in World War II, finishing his enlistment at the 118th General Hospital, a Hopkins center at Fort Meade. Dr. Firor presided over both the Baltimore City Medical Society and the Medical and Chirurgical Faculty. For 15 years he edited *The Yearbook of Radiology.*

1959 - Samuel Whitehouse, M.D. (1895-1981)
An officer in the Canadian Medical Corps during the First World War, Dr. Whitehouse became an internist at Johns Hopkins Hospital. He held staff positions at Sinai Hospital, Hopkins and Greater Baltimore Medical Center. At his retirement he was honored for the 60 years he spent as a cardiologist at Union Memorial Hospital, one of the first Jewish physicians to serve on that hospital's staff.

1960 - Everett S. Diggs, M.D.
Four years after Dr. Diggs received his medical degree from the University of Maryland in 1937, he enlisted and served as a Major in World War II in the Pacific theatre, service for which he received a Presidential Unit Citation and a Bronze Star. He returned to Baltimore and began a long and distinguished career practicing gynecology and female urology at his alma mater, the Hospital for Women of Maryland, Greater Baltimore Medical Center, St. Agnes Hospital, Maryland General Hospital, Baltimore City Hospital, Church Home and Hospital and Union Memorial Hospital. He was an active member of the MedChi Council for many years.

1961 - Charles Wainwright, M.D. (1896-1983)
Dr. Wainwright was a cardiologist at Johns Hopkins Hospital, where he received his medical degree in 1922. He helped establish the first arthritis clinic at Hopkins about 1940.

1962 - R. Carmichael Tilghman, M.D. (1904-1999)
A noted internist at Johns Hopkins Hospital, Dr. Tilghman also achieved local fame by beating off, with an umbrella, an attempted robbery outside the Morris Mechanic Theatre. Before that incident, however, he received his medical degree from Johns Hopkins University and served with the Hopkins Unit in the Pacific in World War II, establishing hospitals in the Fiji Islands and India. Known as a compassionate internist, his specialty was working with pregnant women suffering from cardiac disease. He was an Associate Professor of Medicine at Hopkins, and from 1970-1974 edited the *Johns Hopkins Medical Journal*.

1963 - Harry Robinson, Jr. M.D. (1884-1963)
Beginning his medical career with a degree from the University of Maryland in 1909, Dr. Robinson became Professor of Clinical Dermatology at Hopkins from 1912 until 1955. In addition to articles for professional journals, Dr. Robinson also penned three volumes of verse: *A Few Odd Fancies*, *Jimmy Boy and Other Poems*, and *When Thoughts Go Wandering*.

1964 - Houston S. Everett, M.D. (1901-1975)
Dr. Everett earned his medical degree from Johns Hopkins University in 1925 and was elected to the prestigious Alpha Omega Alpha medical honor fraternity. He went on to become Chair of the Urology Department at the University of Maryland. An expert and textbook author on female urology, Dr. Everett presided over the Baltimore City Medical Society in 1964 and served one term as President of the American Gynecological Club. Dr. J. Donald Woodruff, then Professor of Gynecology at Hopkins, recalled that Dr. Everett was "not only considered one of the finest diagnosticians in the field of female urology, but was an ever-present consultant for the house staff at Hopkins for four decades."

1965 - Samuel Morrison, M.D. (1904-2001)
A gastroenterologist at Union Memorial Hospital and Johns Hopkins Hospital, Dr. Morrison spoke often about the disconnect between modern medical practice and patients' needs. He graduated from the University of Maryland in 1929.

1966 - Arthur George Siwinski, M.D. (1905-1999)
Dr. Siwinski was a surgical oncologist, and in 1966 the President of the Baltimore City Medical Society. He followed that by becoming President of the Medical and Chirurgical Faculty from 1968 to

1969. His medical career began when he received his M.D. degree from the University of Maryland in 1931. During World War II, Dr. Siwinski was an Army medical officer in the southwest Pacific. Dr. Siwinski lectured on dental oncology at the University of Maryland Dental School, and was an Associate Professor at his medical alma mater. He also held staff positions at Mercy, Bon Secours and South Baltimore General Hospitals.

1967 - Harry John Connolly, M.D. (1912-?)
A Georgetown University graduate in 1938, Dr. Connolly served in a surgical hospital during eight campaigns in World War II Europe. Dr. Connolly was Chief of Surgery and President of the Staff at St. Joseph's Hospital

1968 - D. Frank Kaltreider, M.D. (1912-1988)
A voracious reader and excellent hand at bridge, Dr. Kaltreider was on the faculties in obstetrics at both Johns Hopkins University and the University of Maryland, and in charge of the delivery room at Hopkins. From 1962 until 1975 he was Chief of Obstetrics at Hopkins. He taught obstetrics and gynecology at the University of Maryland from 1955 until his retirement, and at Hopkins from 1975-1981. He received his baccalaureate degree from Hopkins, and his medical degree from the University of Maryland in 1937. In 1953 he participated in the birth of one of the children of King Ides and Queen Sadtima of Libya, for which he received a gold watch with the engraved royal shield of Libya. Dr. Kaltreider took his civic duties seriously, working as a volunteer for the March of Dimes and Planned Parenthood. He also established a non-profit Rh testing laboratory in Baltimore.

1969 - Raymond C.V. Robinson, M.D. (1915-1976)
Following the receipt of a degree in pharmacy from the University of Maryland in 1936, Dr. Robinson earned his M.D. degree from the University in 1940. A textbook author, Dr. Robinson compiled a collection of over 8,000 clinical photographs on dermatology. He was a Professor of Dermatology at both Maryland and Hopkins, and Chief of Dermatology at the Greater Baltimore Medical Center and Maryland General Hospital. With his brother, dermatologist Dr. Harry Robinson, Jr.(who was BCMS President in 1963) he wrote *Clinical Dermatology.*

1970 - John N. "Jake" Classen, M.D, (1916-?)
Dr. Classen received his medical degree from Johns Hopkins in 1942 and became Chief of Surgery at Union Memorial Hospital. Dr. Classen was the first Chief of Surgery at Union Memorial, and a noted teacher.

1971 - Philip Franklin Wagley, M.D. (1917-2000)

Dr. Wagley, given his unusually wide experience volunteering in hospital dispensaries and free clinics, advocated organizing physicians nationwide who were concerned about the medical care of the homeless. Dr. Wagley delivered the first lecture on medical ethics at Johns Hopkins University in the fall of 1977, and subsequently directed the school's medical ethics program until his death. In 1995, Hopkins endowed the "Philip F. Wagley Chair in Medical Ethics." He was a founder of the Baltimore City Medical Society Foundation. His private practice patients included one of Baltimore's greatest hypochondriacs, Henry L. Mencken, as well as poet Ogden Nash. Not only was he a prolific medical writer, but Dr. Wagley also published studies on Sherlock Holmes and Dr. Samuel Johnson.

1972 - Edward F. Cotter, M.D (1910-1997)

Dr. Cotter received his medical degree from the University of Maryland in 1935, and remained at the University Hospital as an internist. He was the Director of Medical Education at Maryland General Hospital until his retirement.

"When you hear foot beats behind you, don't expect to see a zebra."

-attributed to Dr. Theodore Woodward
University of Maryland
about 1950

THEODORE E. WOODWARD, M.D.

Actually, Dr. Woodward recalled that the phrase he originally coined was something like "Don't expect to see zebras on Greene Street."* The admonition was uttered in one of his classrooms in the 1940's, and shortly became a standard catchphrase at many medical schools. Greene Street is the location of the University of Maryland School of Medicine, from which he graduated in 1938, and where he held court to rapt medical students until his retirement in 1981. Bernadette Huber Lane, longtime Executive Director of the Baltimore City Medical Society, recalled that it was estimated Dr. Woodward had trained "fully half the physicians in Maryland" by the time he retired.

Dr. Woodward was descended from a distinguished family of physicians. Two generations of Drs. Lewis K. Woodward came first, practicing medicine in Maryland's Carroll County. When the third generation doctor was born, in 1914, his hometown of Westminster was a farm village. He received his bachelors degree at Franklin and Marshall College and went from there to Davidge Hall at the University of Maryland. His wife, Dr. Celeste L. Woodward, was a physician, and each of their three children practice medicine. Upon returning from World War II postings in North Africa, Europe and the Pacific, he entered private practice in Westminster. In 1948, Dr. Woodward was appointed Associate Professor of Medicine at his alma mater, from which he rose to the Chair of the

Department of Medicine. He was Emeritus Professor of Medicine at the University when he retired.

"Life as a teacher of medical students and young physicians, practitioner for patients, and investigator of clinical problems has repaid me much beyond what I have contributed," he wrote in his autobiography *Make Room for Sentiment: A Physician's Story*. In a review of the book, Dr. Philip A. Mackowiak, Professor of Medicine at the University of Maryland, described the story as the chronicle of "a man, who for many years embodied the academic and philosophical essence of the University of Maryland...Few academic institutions are blessed with the good fortune of having a native son rise to such prominence, while devoting his professional life so completely to the betterment of his alma mater."

"When Ted Woodward spoke at a Baltimore City Medical Society meeting," Lane recalled, "we got the largest crowds we ever had."

* "Zebra" is medical slang for a rare, uncommon disease. Dr. Woodward coined it to warn his students against the all-too-common tendency to see an unusual case with every diagnosis.

1973 - Katherine H. Borkovich, M.D. (1915-1994)

The first female President of the Baltimore City Medical Society, Dr. Borkovich was an internist at Johns Hopkins Hospital and a world traveler. She was associated with Johns Hopkins for over 50 years, after receiving her medical degree there in 1939. At Hopkins, she taught pulmonary hypertension, electrocardiology and physical diagnosis (to female students only, as Hopkins classes on topics like this were still gender-segregated). Dr. Borkovich was elected President of the Maryland Society of Internal Medicine in 1964. In 1974 she was named "Internist of the Year" by the American Society of Internal Medicine. Throughout her career, Dr. Borkovich was a major force behind the development of peer review procedures in Maryland, serving on the first Peer Review Committee of the state Faculty, coupling that with dedicated patient advocacy work. Beyond the hospital and the university, she was an avid outdoorswoman and environmentalist. She maintained memberships in the Sierra Club, the Natural History Society of Maryland, the National Audubon Society, the American Forestry Association, the Adirondack Mountain Club and the Fishing Club of America.

1974 - John B. De Hoff, M.D.

Dr. De Hoff's earliest memory of the Baltimore City Medical Society dates to approximately 1928, when his father, who was a practicing physician, took him to a meeting to meet Dr. William H. Welch. "BCMS shared with MedChi the dimly-lighted large lecture room with high-backed, cane-bottomed chairs at the present location on Cathedral Street," he recalled in 1999. "The podium, perhaps still the one in use, was on the room's north wall. Dr. Welch, clearly an old man, sat to the right of the speaker. His audience was attentive, but what he had to say has gone into history, neatly filed there but forgotten." Dr. De Hoff, after receiving his M.D. from Johns Hopkins University in 1939 and his Masters in Public Health in 1967 from the same institution, pursued his own medical career as an internist at Hopkins. In 1965 he joined the Baltimore City Department of Health as Assistant Commissioner for Local Health Services, and he advanced to the Commissioner's position in 1975.

1975 - Douglas Gordon Carroll, M.D. (1915-1997)
Dr. Carroll was President of the Baltimore City Medical Society and a Founding Member and first president of the Baltimore City Medical Society Foundation. He received his medical degree from Johns Hopkins University in 1942 and practiced pulmonary medicine at Hopkins afterwards. During World War II, Dr. Carroll served in the Pacific where he developed an interest in tropical diseases. In 1957 he founded the Department of Rehabilitation and Physical Medicine at Hopkins. Dr. Carroll developed a test for hand function of patients with chronic disabilities. A social activist, he lobbied to secure legislation to meet the crisis in medical malpractice insurance, and advocated for improved health care at the Baltimore City Jail. As a writer, Dr. Carroll edited a monograph of Civil War letters, wrote a history of Baltimore City Hospitals, and a history of the first two centuries of medicine in Maryland, published serially in the *Maryland State Medical Journal*. He was descended from Charles Carroll, Barrister, whose Georgian home "Mount Clare," is a National Historic Landmark in southwest Baltimore.

1976 - Richard L. London, M.D. (1924-1982)
The University of Tennessee granted Dr. London an M.D. degree in 1949, and he went to New Orleans for his internship. Returning to his home, Huntington, West Virginia, he opened his first private practice in 1953. Eventually Dr. London found himself in Baltimore, on the pediatric staffs at University Hospital, St. Agnes Hospital and Greater Baltimore Medical Center. He consulted in pediatric allergies at Mercy Hospital. Dr. London was remembered for his "droll sense of humor," and for his leadership. One of his successors wrote that "His leadership during the malpractice crisis...and during the time of reorganization of the MedChi Council did much to revitalize the BCMS..."

1977 - Ian Russell Anderson, M.D.
Dr. Anderson was Chief Resident, Surgery, at Church Hospital. He received his M.D. degree from the University of Maryland in 1962, and also served on the staffs at Good Samaritan and North Charles General Hospitals.

1978 - Roland Smoot, M.D.
Called a "role model in medicine... for young African Americans," Dr. Smoot became, in 1983, the first African American President of the Medical and Chirurgical Faculty, after having accomplished the same at the Baltimore City Medical Society in 1978. He received his medical degree from Howard University. Dr. Smoot was on the faculty at both Johns Hopkins University and the University of Maryland, eventually rising to Dean of Student Affairs at Hopkins. In addition to being the first African American physician with admitting privileges at Hopkins, he was a staff member at Provident Hospital for many years. He served on the Baltimore Board of Health Services and the Hospital Cost Review Commission.

1979 - Albert Antlitz, M.D.
Dr. Antlitz received his M.D. degree from Georgetown University. A cardiologist at Mercy Hospital, he was President of the Baltimore City Medical Society as well as the state medical Faculty.

1980 - Henry N. Wagner, Jr. M.D.
Dr. Wagner was the Director of the Division of Radiation Health Sciences of the Johns Hopkins School of Public Health, as well as the department of Medicine and Radiology in the Johns Hopkins University school. Dr. Wagner also held a teaching position on the staff at the Hopkins Applied Physics Laboratory. He received his M.D. from Hopkins in 1953 and remained on the staff as Resident of the Osler Medical Service. A founding member of the American Board of Nuclear Medicine, Dr. Wagner served the American Medical Association as a Delegate from Maryland and on the Scientific Affairs Council, and chaired the Association's Section Council on Nuclear Medicine. His contributions to nuclear medicine have brought him countless awards and international recognition. In 1972, Dr. Wagner received the first Vikram Surhabel Gold Medal from the Society of Nuclear Medicine of India, and 1993 brought him the First Annual Society of Nuclear Medicine President's Award. He has been awarded three honorary degrees and is an honorary member of the British Institute of Radiology. The Radiological Society of North America recognized his achievements in 2002.

1981 - Leon Kassel, M.D.
Following his receipt of a medical degree from the University of Virginia Medical School in 1949, Dr. Kassel began a career-long relationship with Sinai Hospital as an intern. After two years in the Air Force, he returned to Sinai in 1954 as Chief Resident in Internal Medicine. While at Sinai he also served as Director of Ambulatory Medical Services, President of the Medical Staff and Chairman of the Medical Executive Committee and edited the *Sinai Hospital Journal*. Dr. Kassel was also an Assistant Professor in the

Department of Epidemiology and Preventive Medicine at the University of Maryland. Dr. Kassel presided over the Baltimore City Medical Society in 1981, and also served as President of the Medical and Chirurgical Faculty.

1982 - Karl H. Weaver, M.D.
Pediatrician Dr. Weaver played a significant role in the implementation of quality improvement steps while Chair of the Department of Pediatrics at the University of Maryland, where he received his medical degree in 1953. Between stints at the University he worked in the Cardiology Department at the National Institutes of Health, and was a post-doctoral research fellow at the Cardiovascular Research Institute of the University of California Medical Center. He served on many committees, was a Board member, and Vice President before assuming the Presidency of the Baltimore City Medical Society in 1982. A member of Alpha Omega Alpha, Dr. Weaver was honored with the Career Research Development Award by the national Institute of Child Health and Human Development.

1983 - Kennard L. Yaffe, M.D.
Dr. Yaffe graduated from the University of Maryland School of Pharmacy in 1934 and followed that degree with an M.D. from the University in 1938. Not only did he preside over the Baltimore City Medical Society, but he held positions at the Medical and Chirurgical Faculty as Chairman of the Drug Committee and a member of the MedChi Council. Before assuming the Society Presidency, Dr. Yaffe accepted positions on many committees, including Peer Review, Health Care Delivery and Finance.

1984 - Raymond M. Atkins, M.D. (1927-1992)
Dr. Atkins's first private practice after completion of his medical degree at the University of Maryland in 1952 was in Chestertown, on Maryland's Eastern Shore. He returned to Baltimore in 1955, entered a surgical residency at Church Home and Hospital and served as Chief of Staff from 1975-1978. In 1989 Dr. Atkins was the President of the Medical and Chirurgical Faculty.

1985 - Elliott Raphael Fishel, M.D. (1919-1985)
Dr. Fishel practiced Industrial Medicine. After returning from a tour of duty in the Army during World War II, he entered Johns Hopkins University and received his medical degree in 1950. He remained at his alma mater as an instructor, and held positions on the staffs of St. Joseph's, Sinai and South Baltimore General Hospitals, as well as Church Home and Hospital. He presided over the Maryland Occupational Medicine Association in 1983, and was President of the Baltimore City Medical Society in 1985. Mid-way through his Presidency of the Baltimore City Medical Society, Dr. Fishel died.

1985/1986 - Gary L. Rosenberg, M.D.
After receiving his M.D. degree from Harvard in1968, internship in Boston and research positions at the National Institutes of Health, Dr. Rosenberg arrived in Baltimore as a Fellow in Allergy and Clinical Immunology at Johns Hopkins University. He has held staff positions at Hopkins and Good Samaritan Hospitals and is head of the Section of Immunology and Allergy at Franklin Square Hospital. Dr. Rosenberg is on the faculty at Johns Hopkins. He was also President of the Maryland Society of Allergy.

1987 - Jose M. Yosuico, M.D.
Immediately after receiving his medical degree from the University of the Philipines in 1953, Dr. Yosuico took his internship at South Baltimore Medical Center and went on to residency at Church Hospital. The internist was President of the state Faculty in addition to presiding over the Baltimore City Medical Society.

1988 - Israel H. Weiner, M.D.
A University of Maryland School of Medicine graduate in 1953, Dr. Weiner is a member of Alpha Omega Alpha. In 1979 he was named President of the Medical Staff of Baltimore County General Hospital, and he was Chairman of the hospital's Board of Physician Quality Assurance. In addition to presiding over the Baltimore City Medical Society, he was President of the Maryland Neurological Society from 1982-1984.

1989 - Hiroshi Nakazawa, M.D.
Dr. Nakazawa received his medical degree in 1956 from Japan's Chiba University, served his internship at the U.S. Naval Hospital in Yokosuka and completed his residency in surgery at St. Agnes and Bon Secours Hospitals. He remained at St. Agnes as an attending physician in the Department of Surgery and Anesthesiology. He became Chief Resident in surgery at St. Agnes in 1961. Dr. Nakazawa holds certification by the American Board of Acupuncture, and has traveled extensively as a lecturer on the topic of medical acupuncture. He presided over the Baltimore City Medical Society in 1989, and from 1997 until 1999 was the President of the Maryland Society of Medical Acupuncture. Dr. Nakazawa was President of the Medical Staff at St. Agnes Hospital (1979-1908) and in 1998 became Secretary of the American Academy of Medical Acupuncture. President Ronald Reagan, in 1987, called Dr. Nakazawa "One of the Ten Most Outstanding Asian Pacific Americans in the United States," and Baltimore Mayor Clarence "Du" Burns declared that December 2, 1988 was "Dr. Hiroshi Nakazawa Day."

1990 - Susan R. Guarnieri, M.D.
After serving as Assistant City Health Commissioner under Dr. John De Hoff, Dr. Guarnieri was appointed to the post of Commissioner in 1984, and served in that position until 1987. She later served as Medical Officer for the Baltimore Gas and Electric Company, and was appointed to the Board of Directors of the Governor's Commission on Women's Health. She is a member of the American Association of Medical Review Officers. Dr. Guarnieri earned her medical degree at Ohio State University in 1966, and her M.P.H. from the Johns Hopkins University School of Hygiene and Public Health in 1969.

1991 - Joseph H. Hooper, Jr., M.D.
Dr. Hooper received his medical degree from Johns Hopkins University School of Medicine in 1954 and after service in the U.S. Navy and residency at the Veterans Administration Hospital at Perry Point, Maryland, he returned to Baltimore and became Chief Surgical Resident at Union Memorial Hospital.

1992 - Allan D. Jensen, M.D.
From 1998-1999, Dr. Jensen was President of the Medical and Chirurgical Faculty, and he presided over the Baltimore City Medical Society in 1992. His medical degree was conferred by Johns Hopkins University in 1968, and he completed a cornea fellowship at the Massachusetts Eye and Ear Infirmary, Harvard, and the Retina Foundation in 1973. Dr. Jensen found himself in Iran as an exchange resident as part of the fellowship, in 1972. Dr. Jensen is an Associate Professor in Ophthalmology at Johns Hopkins University, and as the Baltimore City Medical Society celebrated its centennial in 2004, Dr. Jensen became the President of the American Academy of Ophthalmology.

1993 - Thomas E. Hunt, Jr., M.D.
An orthopedic surgeon, Dr. Hunt is also an amateur historian and an authority on medical history. He graduated from the University of Maryland School of Medicine in 1954, and began his career in 1959 upon completion of his residency in orthopedic surgery at the Johns Hopkins Hospital, where he is now Assistant Professor Emeritus. Dr. Hunt's curricula vitae includes numerous voluntary consultancies: The Johns Hopkins University Limb and Prosthetic Clinic, the Cardinal Shehan Center for the Aging at Stella Maris, and the Allegany County League for Cerebral Palsy and Neuromuscular Disorders, in Cumberland, Maryland. He has presided over the Baltimore City Medical Society (1993) as well as the Maryland Orthopaedic Association (1973-74) and the Lister Society (1995-96). In 1987, Dr. Hunt was honored by membership in the Schmeisser Society (an honorary society of physicians who have given more than 20 years of voluntary service at the Johns

Hopkins School of Medicine). He received the Christophers Spirit Award for services in behalf of the homeless in 1995, and the University of Maryland Distinguished Service Award in 2000.

1994 - Konstantinos G. "Gus" Dritsas, M.D.
Dr. Dritsas received his M.D. degree from the University of Thessalonika, Greece. From 1962 until 1964 he was a Research Fellow at the University of Alberta, in Edmonton, Canada. Dr. Dritsas was Chief of Surgery at the Good Samaritan Hospital from 1976 to 1996. His practice encompassed both general and peripheral vascular surgery.

1995 - Willarda Virginia Edwards, M.D.
Dr. Edwards served as concurrent President of the Baltimore City Medical Society and the local chapter of the National Medical Association (The Monumental City Medical Society) in 1995. She followed her medical degree from the University of Maryland (1977) with a Masters in Business Administration from Loyola College in Maryland in 1999. After four years in the U.S. Navy, at Annapolis (where she was Chief of Internal Medicine) and the Bethesda Naval Hospital, she went into private practice in Baltimore. She has served as a Delegate to the American Medical Association, and on the AMA's Women's Advisory Board. Her most recent appointment is as Director of the Health Division at the NAACP. Dr. Edwards reported that her "professional activities pale in comparison to her volunteer experience as a Big Sister in the Central Maryland Chapter of Big Brothers and Big Sisters." Her dedication to the organization was recognized in 1984 when she was named "Big Sister of the Year," and again in 1991, when she received the Raymond Cain Award. Dr. Edwards has maintained a close relationship with her little sister for over two decades. In 1997 she was named "Woman of the Year in Medicine" by Zeta Phi Beta, a progressive national sorority that provides scholarship assistance through its National Education Foundation and promotes social and civic change. In 2003 she was honored as one of "Maryland's Top 100 Women" by *The Daily Record*. Dr. Edwards was honored in 2004 as a recipient of the Distinguished Women's Award, conferred by the Girl Scouts of Central Maryland. That same year, she became the second woman President of MedChi.

1996 - Murray A. Kalish, M.D.
Dr. Kalish, an Assistant Professor of Anesthesiology and Critical Care Medicine at Johns Hopkins University, became in 1996 the first anesthesiologist to preside over the Baltimore City Medical Society. Much of his career has been spent at the University of Maryland, including a long and distinguished involvement with the R Adams Cowley Shock Trauma Center. Dr. Kalish has served in various positions on both the Advisory and Finance Committees of

the Maryland State Emergency Medical System. He serves on the American Society of Anesthesiologists Board of Directors, and has held the office of Treasurer at the Medical and Chirurgical Faculty. He is a member of the Class of 1973, University of Maryland School of Medicine and was President of the University's Medical Alumni Association. From 1992 through 1995 he was President of the BCMS Foundation. Dr. Kalish is Past President of the Maryland-District of Columbia Society of Anesthesiologists and is on the Board of Directors of the American Society of Anesthesiologists.

1997 - Donald H. Dembo, M.D.
After a year as President of the Medical and Chirurgical Faculty in 1995, Dr. Dembo presided over the Baltimore City Medical Society. He was Chief of Cardiology at Maryland General and Good Samaritan Hospitals and Associate Physician-in-Chief and Vice Chairman of Medicine at Sinai Hospital. Dr. Dembo's baccalaureate degree was earned at Johns Hopkins University, and he received his medical degree from the University of Maryland. He has written extensively in the fields of cardiopulmonary resuscitation and pacemaker technology, with articles appearing in the journals of the Maryland Heart Association, the American Heart Association, the *American Journal of Cardiology* and the *Journal of the American Medical Association*. In 1960, he was awarded a grant by the American Heart Association, Maryland affiliate, to further his study on the application of radioactive materials in the diagnosis of cardiac disease. Dr. Dembo served as Governor for Maryland of the American College of Cardiology, and is on the staff in the Department of Cardiology at Johns Hopkins Hospital. Dr. Dembo's primary interest is in medical education, including serving as education leader in worldwide tours on comparative cardiology. Dr. Dembo was named a "Hero of Medicine" by the AMA.

1998 - Jos Wildman Zebley, III, M.D.
Dr. Zebley was on the staff at the University of Maryland, in Family Practice, and in addition to serving as President of the Baltimore City Medical Society is on the Medical and Chirurgical Faculty Board of Trustees. He is Medical Director of the Center of Health Enhancement at St. Joseph Medical Center and in 1989 was President of the Maryland Academy of Family Physicians. His medical degree was conferred by the University of Maryland in 1976, and he served as resident at the university's Department of Family Medicine. He is Past President of the Maryland Academy of Family Practice, and in 1995 was named "Doctor of the Year" by that organization. In 2003, Dr. Zebley was chosen as one of Baltimore's "Top Docs" by *Baltimore* magazine.

1999 - Beverly A. Collins, M.D.

Dr. Collins earned her M.D. degree from the University of Maryland in 1983 and served for 3 years as a general surgical resident at the University as well as a preventive medicine resident. She received a Masters in Business Administration from Loyola College in Maryland in 1989, and she is Board Certified in Preventive Medicine. She does consulting work in medical quality improvement, patient safety and health care delivery. Dr. Collins is an Adjunct Assistant Professor of Epidemiology and Preventive Medicine at the University of Maryland School of Medicine. She was a Physician Advisor for the Department of Health and Mental Hygiene and Medical Director of Quality Improvement at the Delmarva Foundation for Medical Care.

2000 - John A. Manzari, M.D.

Dr. Manzari is the Director of Medical Education at Maryland General Hospital. He entered the medical profession after receiving his degree from the State University of New York in Buffalo in 1964. Upon graduation, he received the David A. Miller Prize in Medicine from his alma mater and was inducted into Alpha Omega Alpha. He is Senior Vice President of Medical Affairs at Maryland General Hospital. Before serving as the Society's President in 2000, Dr. Manzari presided over the American College of Chest Physicians (New York Chapter) from 1981 until 1982, and the New York State Thoracic Society. He is a Clinical Associate Professor at the University of Maryland. Outside of his medical career, Dr. Manzari is an avid horseman. Among his goals, Dr. Manzari said, is "to own a Triple Crown Winner."

2001 - Reed A. Winston, M.D.

In addition to his medical degree from Howard University in 1978, Dr. Winston holds a PhD conferred by the University of Rochester, Department of Pharmacology and Toxicology. He is Medical Director for the Family Care Practice at Bon Secours Hospital, and in 2003 he became a member of the Nominating Committee of the Board of Directors of CareFirst. Dr. Winston also served as Medical Director of the Emergency Room at Lutheran Hospital and Chairman of Emergency Medicine and Vice President for Medical Affairs at Liberty Medical Center. Dr. Winston is a member of the Legislative Committee of the Medical and Chirurgical Faculty.

2002 - James P.G. "Seamus" Flynn, M.D.
Dr. Flynn received his medical degree from the School of Physicians, Trinity College, Dublin University in 1962. He served his internship in Dublin and then accepted a fellowship in medicine at Johns Hopkins. Dr. Flynn served as Director of the Maryland Institute for Emergency Medical Services System, and Medical Director of Montebello Rehabilitation Hospital. He presided over the Maryland Thoracic Society and has held Board positions at both the Maryland Heart Association and the Provident Adult Day Care Center. Dr. Flynn also served as Vice President of Medical Affairs for the University Specialty and the Lawrence J. Kernan Hospitals. In 2003, Dr. Flynn received the United States Department of Defense Legion of Merit and the Distinguished Service Cross, conferred by the Ministry of Defense of Estonia.

2003 - Eve J. Higginbotham, M.D.
Dr. Higginbotham's professional career has focused on research and treatment of glaucoma, the leading cause of blindness in African Americans. She began her career with bachelors and masters degrees in chemical engineering from the Massachusetts Institute of Technology, and received her M.D. degree from Harvard in 1979. Dr. Higginbotham became Professor and Chair of the Department of Ophthalmology at the University of Maryland School of Medicine in 1994. She was President of the Maryland Society of Eye Physicians in 2000. Dr. Higginbotham has co-edited four books and has been published in over 90 peer-reviewed publications. She served on the Board of Trustees of the American Academy of Ophthalmology, the Advisory Council of the National Eye Institute and the Federal Drug Administration Advisory Panel for Ophthalmic Devices. In 2000, she was inducted into the Institute of Medicine.

2004 - Anil Uberoi, M.D.
Dr. Uberoi became the 101st President of the Baltimore City Medical Society during the Society's centennial year. She received her medical degree from the Lady Harding Medical School, in her native India, and served her residency at the Bronx Lebanon Hospital in New York and the St. Thomas Hospital in Akron, Ohio. From 1995-96 she was Chair of the Department of Medicine at Liberty Health Systems, and she served as the Medical Director of Liberty's Chemical Dependency Unit from 1990-93.

BIBLIOGRAPHY

BOOKS AND PAMPHLETS:

Stephen Ambrose, *Citizen Soldier*, Simon & Schuster, New York, 1997

American Medical Association, *Caring for the Country - A History and Celebration of the First 150 Years of the American Medical Association*, AMA, Chicago, 1997

Baltimore City Department of Public Welfare, *The Baltimore City Health Plan*, Baltimore, 1947

Baltimore City Department of Health, *The Baltimore City Health Plan*, Baltimore, 1954.

Baltimore City Directories, various years 1796 - 1907.

Baltimore City Fire Department, *Municipal Ambulance Service Regulations*, undated pamphlet (probably from about 1927), (Maryland Room, Enoch Pratt Free Library, Baltimore)

"Baltimore City Medical Society", undated brochure, Baltimore City Medical Society, Village of Cross Keys, Baltimore (Maryland Room, Enoch Pratt Free Library, Baltimore)

Baltimore City Medical Society, *The Sad Case of Waiting Room Willie*, 1952, with correspondence referring to the book including two undated press releases (Maryland Room, Enoch Pratt Free Library, Baltimore)

Baltimore City Medical Society Committee on Public Education, "Subjects for Talks", November 30, 1953 (Maryland Room, Enoch Pratt Free Library, Baltimore)

Baltimore City Medical Society Minutes Book, April, 1904 - November, 1915, 1 bound volume, collection of the Baltimore City Medical Society

Baltimore City Medical Society Minutes Book, December, 1915 - December, 1919, 1 bound volume, collection of the Baltimore City Medical Society

Baltimore City Medical Society Minutes Book, December, 1919 - December, 1931, 1 ring binder, collection of the Baltimore City Medical Society

Baltimore City Medical Society Minutes Book, January, 1932 - December, 1942, 1 ring binder, collection of the Baltimore City Medical Society

Baltimore City Medical Society Minutes Book, January, 1943 - December, 1949, 1 ring binder, collection of the Baltimore City Medical Society

Baltimore City Medical Society Minutes Books, 1950-1971, 12 volumes in ring binders, collection of the Baltimore City Medical Society

Baltimore City Medical Society Newsletters, 1972-2004, 11 volumes in ring binders, collection of Baltimore City Medical Society

Baltimore City Medical Society, BCMS Reports, 1990-2003, 1 volume in ring binder, collection of Baltimore City Medical Society

Baltimore Medical Association Minutes, 1869-1874, 1891-1897, 3 volumes. Medical and Chirurgical Faculty collection Maryland Historical Society MS 3000 #122

Baltimore Medical Association, *Constitution and By-Laws of the Baltimore Medical Association*, Frederick A. Hanzsche, 234 Baltimore Street, Baltimore, 1866

Katherine Traver Barkley, *The Ambulance*, Exposition Press, Hicksville NY, 1978

A. Walker Bingham, *The Snake-Oil Syndrome*, A. Walter Bingham, New York, 1993

W. Brinton, M.D., *Transactions of the Medical and Chirurgical Faculty, 1881, 1882*, J. W. Borst and Company, Baltimore, 1881, G. Lane Taneyhill, "Historical Sketches of the Medical Societies of Baltimore, Md. from 1730 to 1880", pgs. 283-297. This essay was read by Dr. Taneyhill on the occasion of the Commemoration of the Sesquicentennial of the City of Baltimore, October 13, 1880.

W.F. Bynum and Roy Porter, *Companion Encyclopedia of the History of Medicine* (2 volumes), Routledge and Company, London, 1994

Douglas Carroll, M.D., "History of the Baltimore City Hospitals," *Maryland Medical Journal* (vol. 15), Baltimore, 1966.

Samuel Claggett Chew, M.D., *Addresses on Several Occasions*, the Deutch Company, Baltimore, 1906.

Eugene Fauntleroy Cordell, M.D., *The Importance of the Study of the History of Medicine, An Address delivered on the 150th Anniversary of the Medical and Chirurgical Faculty of the State of Maryland, April 27, 1904*, Killiam and Geyer Printers, Baltimore, 1904

Eugene Fauntleroy Cordell, M.D., *University of Maryland, 1807-1907 - Its History, Influence, Equipment and Characteristics with Biographical Sketches and Portraits of its Founders, Benefactors, Regents, Faculty and Alumni, Vol. I*, Lewis Publishing Company, New York, Chicago, 1907.

Thomas S. Cullen, *Early Medicine in Maryland* (booklet with no publication information or date, in the library of the Maryland Historical Society)

Dieter Cunz, *The Maryland Germans - A History*, Kennikat Press, Port Washington NY, 1972

Denney, Robert E., *Civil War Medicine - Care & Comfort of the Wounded*, Sterling Publishing Co., Inc., New York, 1995

Steven B. Duke and Albert C. Gross, *America's Longest War, Rethinking Our Tragic Crusade Against Drugs*, G.P. Putnam's Sons, New York, 1994

East Baltimore Medical Association, *Constitution and By-Laws of the (East) Baltimore Medical Association*, Steam Press Fred. A. Hanzsche, No. 106 Baltimore Street, Baltimore, 1871 (Note: This is actually a copy of the 1866 Baltimore Medical Association By-Laws, altered in pencil as a draft copy of proposed By-Laws for the East Baltimore group. The booklet was given to the Medical and Chirurgical Faculty of Maryland Library by Dr. A. Erich, the first President of the East Baltimore Medical Association, or the Medical and Surgical Association of Baltimore as it came to be formally known).

John C. French, *A Brief History of the Medical and Chirurgical Faculty of Maryland*, Waverly Press, Baltimore, 1949

Suzanne Ellery Greene, *An Illustrated History of Baltimore*, Windsor Publications, Woodland Hills, California, 1980

Mary Ellen Hayward and Charles Belfoure, *The Baltimore Rowhouse*, Princeton Architectural Press, New York, 1999

Thomas E. Hunt, Jr. M.D., "History of 819 Park Avenue", Baltimore City Medical Society, Baltimore, 1982.

A.N. Marquis Company, *Who was Who in America*, Chicago, 1963.

The Medical Alumni Association of the University of Maryland, Inc., *Davidge Hall*, Baltimore (undated pamphlet).

Henry Louis Mencken and George Jean Nathan, *The American Credo*, Alfred A. Knopf, New York, 1920

Monumental City Medical Society, *Pioneers in Medicine Awards Dinner*, 2001 and 2003

National Biographical Publishing Company, *The Biographical Cyclopedia of Representative Men of Maryland and the District of Columbia*, Baltimore, 1879.

David Nichols, *Ernie's War - The Best of Ernie Pyle's World War II Dispatches*, Random House, New York, 1986

Sherry H. Olson, *Baltimore, The Building of an American City*, Johns Hopkins University Press, Baltimore and London, 1980

Hamilton Owens, *Baltimore on the Chesapeake*, Doubleday Doran and Company, Garden City NY, 1941

John R. Quinan, M.D., *Medical Annals of Baltimore*, Press of Isaac Friedenwald, Baltimore, 1884.

Edward T. Schultz, *History of Freemasonry in Maryland*, J. Medairy and Company, Baltimore, 1888

Jane Elliot Sewell, *Medicine in Maryland, the Practice and Profession, 1799-1999*, Johns Hopkins University Press, Baltimore and London, 1999

Russell S. Sobel, *Public Health and the Placebo: The Legacy of the 1906 Pure Food and Drug Act*, photocopy of ms. In Maryland Room, Enoch Pratt Free Library, no date or publisher noted

NEWSPAPERS AND MAGAZINES:

Various issues of the *Maryland Journal and Baltimore Daily Advertiser*, 1785-1790
"Medical Society Elects Dr. R. P. Bay", *Sun*, Dec (undeciph), 1936, Baltimore
"Opinions Reported on Health Trends," *Sun*, Baltimore, April 4, 1937
"Group Advocates State Provide Medical Care for Indigent in the Counties," *Sun*, Baltimore, April 20, 1944
Louis J. O'Donnell, "Legislature Gets O'Conor Medical Plan," *Sun*, Baltimore, January 16, 1945
"City Medical Group Plans Meetings", *Evening Sun*, Baltimore, March 4, 1947
"Medical Publicity Group Formed", *Evening Sun*, August 5, 1949, Baltimore
Virginia Tracy, "Medical Society Auxiliary Formed," *Evening Sun*, Baltimore, March 6, 1950
"Medical Group To Get Award", *Sun*, April 19, 1950, Baltimore
"Medical Society To Get Award", *Evening Sun*, April 21, 1950, Baltimore
"Deserved Recognition", *Evening Sun*, April 22, 1950, Baltimore
"Medical Society Receives Honor", *Sun*, April 22, 1950, Baltimore
"24 Hour Service for Emergency Doctors Starts," *Sun*, Baltimore, May 25, 1950
"Emergency Medical Service Handles 91 Calls in 17 Days," *Evening Sun*, Baltimore, May 26, 1950
"Druggists May Assist in Emergency Plan," *Evening Sun*, Baltimore, June 29, 1950
"Chairmen Named in Medical Auxiliary," *Evening Sun*, Baltimore, September 22, 1950
"351 Doctors Take Part in Emergency Service," *Evening Sun*, Baltimore, April 30, 1952
"Doctors Here Study Sliding Scale of Fees", *Sun*, October 27, 1952, Baltimore
"Doctors Veto Plan For Fee Cooperative", *Sun*, January 12, 1953, Baltimore
"City Medical Society Rejects Dr. Ruth Bleier as a Member", *Sun*, March 21, 1953, Baltimore
"Dr. Bleier to Fight Bar by Doctors," *Sun*, Baltimore, March 21, 1953
Frank Henry, "300 Years of Maryland Medicine", *Sun*, Baltimore, November 15, 1953
"Doctors' Speakers Bureau Formed", *Evening Sun*, March 9, 1954, Baltimore
Jeanne H. Sargeant, "Emergency Calls Will be Screened," *Evening Sun*, Baltimore, May 22, 1962

Peter Young, "Dr. Helen Taussig Reflects on Career as Pediatrician," *Evening Sun*, Baltimore, June 19, 1963

Huntington Williams, M.D., "Osler and Welch - Founders of Modern American Public Health," *Baltimore Health News*, Baltimore City Health Department, Baltimore, August, 1963.

Thomas T. Fenton, "Doctors Vote $140,000 for Fight on Bill," *Sun*, Baltimore, February 21, 1965

Thomas T. Fenton, "City Doctors Reject Levy on Medicare," *Sun*, Baltimore, April 3, 1965

Thomas T. Fenton, "Doctors Get Boycott Plan on Medicare," *Sun*, Baltimore, August 20, 1965

Thomas T. Fenton, "City Medical Society Admits 'Anti-Medicare' Fee Unrest," *Sun*, Baltimore, September 24, 1965

Jonathan Cottin, "Connolly Would Be Rift Healer", *Evening Sun*, January 11, 1966, Baltimore

"Kaltreider Only Nomination for Medical Society Head", *Sun*, November 7, 1966, Baltimore

Frederick P. McGehan, "The Medical Society Probes Itself", *Sun*, December 17, 1968

Roger Twigg, "City's ambulances still free at 50," *Sun*, Baltimore, June 25, 1977

Katherine A. Harvey, "Practicing Medicine at the Baltimore Almshouse," *Maryland Historical Society Quarterly*, Baltimore, Fall, 1979

Charles C. Euchner, "The Politics of Urban Expansion: Baltimore and the Sewerage Question," *Maryland Historical Society Quarterly*, Maryland Historical Society, Baltimore, Fall, 1991

Joseph M. Miller, M.D., "The Baltimore General Dispensary: withhold not thy hand", *Maryland Medical Journal*, July, 1995

Peggy Haile McPhillips and Benjamin H. Trask, "The Darker Side of Commerce: Yellow Fever in the Chesapeake Bay", *Chesapeake Bay Maritime Museum Quarterly*, St. Michaels, Maryland, Winter 2003-2004

James M. Kramon, "Doctors Reach a Crisis Point," *Sun*, Baltimore, January 11, 2004

Associated Press, "Doctors to Rally for Malpractice Reform," *Sun*, Baltimore, January 19, 2004

Scott E. Maizel, "Time for a Change," *Sun*, Baltimore, January 21, 2004

Meredith Cohn, "Physicians Protest Cost of Insurance," *Sun*, Baltimore, January 22, 2004

Peter Kumpa, "Baltimore's Medical History: Years of Controversy and Commitment", *Sun*, Baltimore, undated clipping in the vertical files of the Maryland Historical Society library

Frederick P. McGehan, "Negro Group Drawing New Care Plans," *Sun*, Baltimore, undated clipping

"The Girl with the Lamp," Library of Congress card catalog file # fi 54000021

WEBSITES:

http://www.theaha.org/Projects/GIroundtable/Health/Health4.htm
  website of the American Hospital Association
http://www.haciendapub.com/annis.html
  "Towards Socialized Medicine", Edward R. Annis M.D., 2002
  (Dr. Annis is a past president of the AMA)
http://www.bcmsdocs.org
  Baltimore City Medical Society
http://www.bcbs.com
  Who We Are - The Blue Cross Blue Shield System
http://www.citypaper.com
  Website of the *City Paper*, Baltimore
http://history1900s.about.com/library/weekly/aa062900c.htm
  The History Net - 20th Century History
http://hnn.us/articles/1583.html
  "What is Medicare?", Will Mallon, 2003
http://www.mdhistoryonline
  Maryland history website
http://www.ci.new-bedford.ma.us/PSAFETY/EMGSRVS/hstry
  State of Massachusetts Emergency Medical Service history
http://www.nmanet.org
  Website of the National Medical Association
http://www.civilwarmed.org
  National Museum of Civil War Medicine
http://www.cr.nps.gov/abpp/battles
  The Battle of Cedar Mountain
  National Park Service, Cedar Mountain Battlefield
http://www.medinfo.ufl.edu/other/histmed/lemire
  Online slide show, history of emergency services
http://www.sannet.gov/fireandems/911/emshist.shtml
  San Diego, California, Emergency Medical Service history
http://www.civilwarhome.com
  Civil War Potpourri
  "Shotgun's" Home of the American Civil War
http://www.civilwarhome.com/medicinehistory
  Caring for the Men - The History of Civil War Medicine
http://www.scdhec.net/hr/ems/history
  South Carolina Emergency Services
http://www.tdh.state.tx.us/hcqs/ems/StratPrepHistory
  Texas Emergency Medical Services history
http://www.trumanlibrary.org
  Website of the Truman Presidential Museum and Library
http://www.cl.utoledo.edu/canaday/quackery/quack
  From Quackery to Bacteriology - Medicine in the Civil War
  University of Toledo Libraries

SPECIAL ACKNOWLEDGMENTS

To Richard Behles, of the University of Maryland Medical School Library, for getting this project started on the right foot,

To those members of the Baltimore City Medical Society who reviewed and edited the manuscript during its progress, and for providing insight into the Society's recent history, including Drs. Donald Dembo, John De Hoff, Beverly Collins, Thomas Hunt, Eve Higginbotham, Tyler Cymet, Murray Kalish, Albert Jensen, Timothy Baker, Gaylord L. Clark and Sheldon Goldgeier,

To Judge John Carroll Byrnes, distinguished Judge and State Senator, and President of the Baltimore City Historical Society for reviewing the manuscript with the eyes of a jurist and an historian,

To the staff in the Maryland Room at the Enoch Pratt Free Library for assisting with research using the library's Maryland vertical file archives,

To Bernadette Huber Lane, Carol E. Mills and Lisa B. Williams for taking their time to endure interviews and answer questions,

To Drs. Thomas Hunt, John De Hoff, and Roland Smoot for answering our questions during interviews, and

To the staff of the Maryland Historical Society Library.

About the Authors...

Pat and Ron Pilling divide their time between Maryland's Eastern Shore and downtown Baltimore. An educator and researcher, Pat is the Historian at the Star Spangled Banner Flag House and War of 1812 Museum in Baltimore. She earned BS and MEd degrees at Towson University. Ron has written extensively about local and regional history, both for magazines and a series of travel and promotional books about Baltimore, Annapolis and Maryland. He received a BS degree from the University of Maryland and an MBA from Morgan University. In addition, Pat is an avid organic gardener and Ron is an environmental activist for Maryland's seashore and coastal bays.

BALTIMORE CITY COMMISSIONERS OF HEALTH
1793 - 2004

1793-1794	John Worthington, M.D.
	John Ross, M.D.
	Thomas Drysdalle, M.D.
1795-1796	Records unavailable
1797	Jeramiah Yellott, M.D.
	Emanuel Kent, M.D.
	James Edwards, M.D.
	Joseph Townsend, M.D.
	Adam Fonerden, M.D.
	Elias Ellicott, M.D.
	John Steele, M.D.
	Thomas Tenant, M.D.
	James Beeman, M.D.
1798	William Winchester, M.D.
	Joseph Townsend, M.D.
	Michael Diffenderfer, M.D.
	John E. Reefe, M.D.
	William C. Goldsmith, M.D.
	John Dalrymple, M.D.
	Levin Hall, M.D.
	James Biays, M.D.
	Benjamin Thomas, M.D.
1799	Records unavailable
1800	Adam Fonerden, M.D.
	Joseph Townsend, M.D.
1801-1803	Records unavailable
1804-1805	Alexander Ashton, M.D.
1806-1808	Records unavailable
1809	John Crawford, M.D.
1810	William Stewart, M.D.
1811	Records unavailable
1812	Alexander Ashton, M.D.
1813	Records unavailable
1814-1818	William Stewart, M.D.
1819-1821	Records unavailable
1822	James Martin, M.D.
	Peter Foy, M.D.
	William Reaney, M.D.
1823	Records unavailable
1824	Peter Foy, M.D.
	Thomas S. Sheppard, M.D.
	John Dukehart, M.D.
1825-1826	Peter Foy, M.D.
	William Reaney, M.D.
	Thomas S. Sheppard, M.D.
1827-1832	Thomas S. Sheppard, M.D.
	Jacob Deems, M.D.
	Peter Foy, M.D.

1833-1838	Peter Foy, M.D.
	Jacob Deems, M.D.
	William Steuart, M.D.
1839	Thomas E. Bond, M.D.
	Peter Foy, M.D.
	Jacob Small, M.D.
1840	Charles S. Davis, M.D.
	Peter Foy, M.D.
	Jacob Deems, M.D.
1841-1843	Richard Marley, M.D.
	George Rodenmayer, M.D.
	Isaac Glass, M.D.
1844	John N. Murphy, M.D.
	George A. Davis, M.D.
	John Ijams, M.D.
1845-1846	William T. Leonard, M.D.
	D.H. Lawrence, M.D.
	James Peregoy, M.D.
1847-1848	William T. Leonard, M.D.
	James Peregoy, M.D.
	Edward L. Chaisty, M.D.
	D.H. Lawrence, M.D.
1849	John F. Monmonier, M.D.*
	J.F.C. Hadel, M.D.
	Edward J. Chaisty, M.D.
1850	J.F.C. Hadel, M.D.
1851-1852	Charles H. Bradford, M.D.
1853-1854	Charles A. Leas, M.D.
1855-1860	J.W. Houck, M.D.
1861	Charles H. Bradford, M.D.
1862-1865	Samuel T. Knight, M.D.
1866-1867	Gerard E. Morgan, M.D.*
1868-1871	Milton N. Taylor, M.D.
1872	George Benson, M.D.
1873-1881	James A. Steuart, M.D.*
1882-1883	George Benson, M.D.
1884-1889	James A. Steuart, M.D.*
1890	George A. Rohe, M.D.
1891-1897	James F. McShane, M.D.
1898-1899	C. Hampson Jones, M.D.*
1900-1912	James Bosley, M.D.
1913-1914	Nathan R. Gorter, M.D.
1915-1918	John D. Blake, M.D.*
1919-1932	C. Hampson Jones, M.D.*
1933-1961	Huntington Williams, M.D.
1962-1974	Robert E. Farber, M.D.
1975-1983	John B. De Hoff, M.D.*
1984-1986	Susan R. Guarnieri, M.D.*
1987-1989	Maxie T. Collier, M.D.
1990-1991	Elias A. Dorsey, M.P.H. (Acting)
1992-Present	Peter L. Beilenson, M.D.

Note: The Department of Health was reorganized often, and the numbers and terms of Commissioners changed frequently.

*Known to have been the President of a Baltimore medical society